Vasectomy and Vasectomy Reversal: Important Issues

Guest Editors

JAY I. SANDLOW, MD
HARRIS M. NAGLER, MD, FACS

UROLOGIC CLINICS
OF NORTH AMERICA

www.urologic.theclinics.com

August 2009 • Volume 36 • Number 3

SAUNDERS an imprint of ELSEVIER, Inc.

W.B. SAUNDERS COMPANY
A Division of Elsevier Inc.

1600 John F. Kennedy Blvd. ● Suite 1800 ● Philadelphia, PA 19103-2899

http://www.theclinics.com

UROLOGIC CLINICS OF NORTH AMERICA Volume 36, Number 3
August 2009 ISSN 0094-0143, ISBN-13: 978-1-4377-1278-0, ISBN-10: 1-4377-1278-9

Editor: Kerry Holland
Developmental Editor: Donald Mumford

Urologic Clinics of North America (ISSN 0094-0143) is published quarterly by Elsevier Inc., 360 Park Avenue South, New York, NY 10010-1710. Months of issue are February, May, August, and November. Business and Editorial Offices: 1600 John F. Kennedy Blvd., Suite 1800, Philadelphia, PA 19103-2899. Periodicals postage paid at New York, NY and additional mailing offices. Subscription prices are $269.00 per year (US individuals), $429.00 per year (US institutions), $308.00 per year (Canadian individuals), $526.00 per year (Canadian institutions), $383.00 per year (foreign individuals), and $526.00 per year (foreign institutions). Foreign air speed delivery is included in all *Clinics* subscription prices. All prices are subject to change without notice. **POSTMASTER:** Send address changes to *Urologic Clinics of North America*, Elsevier Periodicals Customer Service, 11830 Westline Industrial Drive, St. Louis, MO 63146. Customer Service: 1-800-654-2452 (US). From outside the United States, call 1-314-453-7041. Fax: 1-314-453-5170. E-mail: JournalsCustomerServiceusa@elsevier.com (for print support) and JournalsOnlineSupport-usa@elsevier.com (for online support).

Reprints. For copies of 100 or more, of articles in this publication, please contact the Commercial Reprints Department, Elsevier Inc., 360 Park Avenue South, New York, New York 10010-1710. Tel.: 212-633-3813; Fax: 212-462-1935; E-mail: reprints@elsevier.com.

Urologic Clinics of North America is covered in MEDLINE/PubMed (*Index Medicus*), *Excerpta Medica, Current Contents/Clinical Medicine, Science Citation Index,* and *ISI/BIOMED.*

Printed and bound in the United Kingdom

Transferred to Digital Print 2011

Contributors

GUEST EDITORS

JAY I. SANDLOW, MD
Professor of Urology and Vice Chairman, Department of Urology; Department of Obstetrics and Gynecology, Medical College of Wisconsin, Milwaukee, Wisconsin

HARRIS M. NAGLER, MD, FACS
Interim President and Chair, Sol and Margaret Berger Department of Urology, Beth Israel Medical Center; Chief of Academic Affairs/Graduate Medical Education, Beth Israel Medical Center; and Professor of Urology, The Albert Einstein College of Medicine of Yeshiva University, New York, New York

AUTHORS

CHRISTOPHER E. ADAMS, MD
Resident, Department of Urology, University of Iowa, Iowa City, Iowa

KEVIN S. ART, MD
Department of Urology, University of Kansas Medical Center, Kansas City, Kansas

MARK A. BARONE, DVM, MS
Senior Medical Associate, Programs Division, EngenderHealth, New York, New York

RICHARD C. BENNETT, MD
Fellow, Scott Department of Urology, Division of Male Reproductive Medicine and Surgery, Baylor College of Medicine, Houston, Texas

ROBERT E. BRANNIGAN, MD
Associate Professor, Department of Urology, Northwestern University, Feinberg School of Medicine, Chicago, Illinois

ANEES A. FAZILI, MD
Department of Urology, Northwestern University, Feinberg School of Medicine, Chicago, Illinois

MARC GOLDSTEIN, MD, FACS
Mathew P. Hardy Distinguished Professor of Reproductive Medicine, Department of Urology, and Surgeon-in-Chief, Male Reproductive Medicine and Surgery, Cornell Institute for Reproductive Medicine, New York-Presbyterian Hospital/Weill Cornell Medical Center, Weill Cornell Medical College; and Senior Scientist, The Population Council, Center for Biomedical Research, New York, New York

HOWARD JUNG, MD
Chief Resident, Sol and Margaret Berger Department of Urology, Philips Ambulatory Care Centre, Beth Israel Medical Center, New York, New York

ANDREW I. KAPLAN, Esq
Aaronson, Rappaport, Feinstein & Deutsch, LLP, New York, New York

HOWARD H. KIM, MD
Fellow in Male Reproductive Medicine and Microsurgery, Department of Urology, Cornell Institute for Reproductive Medicine, New York-Presbyterian Hospital/Weill Cornell Medical Center, Weill Cornell Medical College; and Research Fellow, The Population Council, Center for Biomedical Research, New York, New York

TOBIAS S. KÖHLER, MD, MPH
Division of Urology, Southern Illinois University,
Springfield, Illinois

MICHEL LABRECQUE, MD, PhD
Professeur titulaire, Département de médecine
familiale et de medicine d'urgence, Université
Laval, Centre de recherché du CHUQ, Hôpital
Saint-François d'Assise, Québec, Québec,
Canada

LARRY I. LIPSHULTZ, MD
Chief, Division of Male Reproductive Medicine
and Surgery, Professor, Scott Department of
Urology, Lester and Sue Smith Chair in
Reproductive Medicine, Baylor College
of Medicine, Houston, Texas

HARRIS M. NAGLER, MD, FACS
Interim President and Chair, Sol and Margaret
Berger Department of Urology, Beth Israel
Medical Center; Chief of Academic Affairs/
Graduate Medical Education, Beth Israel
Medical Center; and Professor of Urology, The
Albert Einstein College of Medicine of Yeshiva
University, New York, New York

AJAY K. NANGIA, MBBS
Associate Professor, Department of Urology,
and Clinical Director of Andrology, Male
Infertility, and Microsurgery, University of
Kansas Medical Center, Kansas City, Kansas

JOHN M. PILE, MPH
Senior Advisor, The RESPOND Project,
Programs Division, EngenderHealth,
New York, New York

JAY A. RAPPAPORT, Esq
Aaronson, Rappaport, Feinstein & Deutsch,
LLP, New York, New York

PAUL ROBB, MD
Assistant Professor, Department of Obstetrics
and Gynecology, Medical College of
Wisconsin, Milwaukee, Wisconsin

JON A. RUMOHR, MD
Fellow, Scott Department of Urology,
Division of Male Reproductive Medicine
and Surgery, Baylor College of Medicine,
Houston, Texas

JAY I. SANDLOW, MD
Professor of Urology and Vice Chairman,
Department of Urology; Department of
Obstetrics and Gynecology, Medical College of
Wisconsin, Milwaukee, Wisconsin

YEFIM R. SHEYNKIN, MD, FACS
Associate Professor, Department of Urology
and Director, Male Infertility and
Microsurgery, Health Science Center,
State University of New York at Stony Brook,
Stony Brook, New York

DAVID C. SOKAL, MD
Senior Scientist, Behavioral and Biomedical
Research Department, Family Health
International, Research Triangle Park,
North Carolina

MOSHE WALD, MD
Assistant Professor, Department of Urology,
University of Iowa, Iowa City, Iowa

Contents

> Vasectomy is a safe and effective procedure for permanent contraception. Vasectomy is 30 times less likely to fail and 20 times less likely to have postoperative complications than its gynecologic counterpart. Complications from vasectomy are rare and minor in nature. Immediate risks include infection, hematoma, and pain. Complications seldom lead to hospitalization or aggressive medical management. Technique is surgeon dependent; however, certain techniques, such as fascial interposition, seem to decrease rates of vasectomy failure. Despite myriad vasectomy techniques, failure rates are less than those seen with tubal ligation. Available data suggest that vasectomized men do not seem at increased risk for immune-complex diseases.

> Vasectomy is widely regarded as a safe method of contraception, but over the years there have been many reports suggesting putative health risks associated with the procedure. Concerns over the possible association of vasectomy with a number of medical conditions, including cardiovascular disease, testicular cancer, prostate cancer, psychologic distress, and a variety of immune complex–mediated disease processes have been reported. Most recently, a manuscript from the neurology literature has described an association between vasectomy and primary progressive aphasia, a rare variety of frontotemporal dementia. This article reviews the literature surrounding each of these purported health concerns. Because the ultimate findings have important ramifications for both informed consent of vasectomy patients and for public health, the reported health risks in question should be critically evaluated.

> This article explores why the national court system has seen a steady influx of claims alleging practitioners' failure properly to perform vasectomy or ensure sterilization and the manner in which that influx has caused physicians to reassess their methods of practicing medicine in an increasingly litigious environment and make the appropriate and necessary accommodations. Through their experiences as medical malpractice litigators and through the analysis of reported cases, national jury verdicts, and insurance claims made and paid in lawsuits arising from claims regarding the performance of vasectomy, the authors enlighten the reader as to the legal theories and hurdles applicable to such claims and the medical theories most often elucidated and litigated by the patients who bring them. Also offered are suggestions as to the manner in which the practitioner may be proactive in both preventing and defending exposure to malpractice litigation.

> Vasectomy reversal has come a long way since the first anastomosis of the vas deferens and epididymis. Although its history is not as politically charged as that of vasectomy, the progress of reversal surgery has had its share of brilliant discoveries and missteps. In the early part of the twentieth century, vasovasostomy and

vasoepididymostomy were esoteric procedures, but by the 1970s, a majority of urologists had some experience with reversal surgery. With the advent of microsurgical technique, reversal surgery has become once more a specialist's undertaking. The history of vasectomy reversal is an excellent case study in the evolution of surgery.

GOAL STATEMENT

The goal of *Urologic Clinics of North America* is to keep practicing urologists and urology residents up to date with current clinical practice in urology by providing timely articles reviewing the state of the art in patient care.

ACCREDITATION

The *Urologic Clinics of North America* is planned and implemented in accordance with the Essential Areas and Policies of the Accreditation Council for Continuing Medical Education (ACCME) through the joint sponsorship of the University of Virginia School of Medicine and Elsevier. The University of Virginia School of Medicine is accredited by the ACCME to provide continuing medical education for physicians.

The University of Virginia School of Medicine designates this educational activity for a maximum of 12 *AMA PRA Category 1 Credits*™ for each issue, 60 credits per year. Physicians should only claim credit commensurate with the extent of their participation in the activity.

The American Medical Association has determined that physicians not licensed in the US who participate in this CME activity are eligible for a maximum of 12 *AMA PRA Category 1 Credits*™ for each issue, 60 credits per year.

Credit can be earned by reading the text material, taking the CME examination online at: http://www.theclinics.com/home/cme, and completing the evaluation. After taking the test, you will be required to review any and all incorrect answers. Following completion of the test and evaluation, your credit will be awarded and you may print your certificate.

FACULTY DISCLOSURE/CONFLICT OF INTEREST

The University of Virginia School of Medicine, as an ACCME accredited provider, endorses and strives to comply with the Accreditation Council for Continuing Medical Education (ACCME) Standards of Commercial Support, Commonwealth of Virginia statutes, University of Virginia policies and procedures, and associated federal and private regulations and guidelines on the need for disclosure and monitoring of proprietary and financial interests that may affect the scientific integrity and balance of content delivered in continuing medical education activities under our auspices.

The University of Virginia School of Medicine requires that all CME activities accredited through this institution be developed independently and be scientifically rigorous, balanced and objective in the presentation/discussion of its content, theories and practices.

All authors/editors participating in an accredited CME activity are expected to disclose to the readers relevant financial relationships with commercial entities occurring within the past 12 months (such as grants or research support, employee, consultant, stock holder, member of speakers bureau, etc.). The University of Virginia School of Medicine will employ appropriate mechanisms to resolve potential conflicts of interest to maintain the standards of fair and balanced education to the reader. Questions about specific strategies can be directed to the Office of Continuing Medical Education, University of Virginia School of Medicine, Charlottesville, Virginia.

The faculty and staff of the University of Virginia Office of Continuing Medical Education have no financial affiliations to disclose.

The authors/editors listed below have identified no professional or financial affiliations for themselves or their spouse/partner:
Christopher E. Adams, MD; Kevin S. Art, MD; Mark A. Barone, DVM, MS; Richard C. Bennett, MD; Robert E. Brannigan, MD; Kerry K. Holland (Acquisitions Editor); Anees Ahmed Fazili, MD; Howard Jung, MD; Andrew I. Kaplan, Esq.; Howard H. Kim, MD; Tobias S. Köhler, MD, MPH; Harris M. Nagler, MD, FACS (Guest Editor); Ajay K. Nangia, MBBS; John M. Pile, MPH; Jay A. Rappaport, Esq.; Paul Robb, MD; Jon A. Rumohr, MD; Jay I. Sandlow, MD (Guest Editor); Yefim R. Sheynkin, MD, FACS; William Steers, MD (Test Author); and Moshe Wald, MD.

The authors/editors listed below identified the following professional or financial affiliations for themselves or their spouse/partner:
Marc Goldstein, MD, FACS serves on the Advisory Committee for Therologix.
Michel Lacrecque, MD, PhD is an industry funded research/investigator for and owns stock in Contravac, Inc.
Larry I. Lipschultz, MD is an industry funded research/investigator for Allegran and Auxilium, is a consultant for Auxilium and Pfizer, and serves on the Speakers Bureau for AMS, Auxilium, and Lilly.
David C. Sokal, MD is a consultant for Twin Star Medical/Shepherd Medical and is employed by Family Health International.

Disclosure of Discussion of Non-FDA Approved Uses for Pharmaceutical Products and/or Medical Devices.
The University of Virginia School of Medicine, as an ACCME provider, requires that all faculty presenters identify and disclose any off-label uses for pharmaceutical and medical device products. The University of Virginia School of Medicine recommends that each physician fully review all the available data on new products or procedures prior to clinical use.

TO ENROLL

To enroll in the Urologic Clinics of North America Continuing Medical Education program, call customer service at 1-800-654-2452 or visit us online at: www.theclinics.com/home/cme. The CME program is available to subscribers for an additional fee of $195.00.

Urologic Clinics of North America

THE CLINICS ARE NOW AVAILABLE ONLINE!

Access your subscription at:
www.theclinics.com

Preface

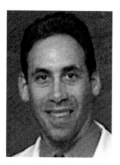 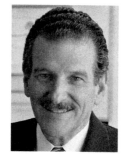

Jay I. Sandlow, MD   Harris M. Nagler, MD, FACS
Guest Editors

Vasectomy is a safe and effective method of contraception that should be viewed as permanent. In the United States, it is employed by nearly 11% of all married couples and is performed on approximately one-half million men each year. Thus, vasectomies are carried out more often than any other urologic surgical procedure. Worldwide, however, far fewer vasectomies are performed than female sterilizations by tubal ligation, even though vasectomy is less expensive and is associated with less morbidity and mortality than tubal ligation. This apparent underutilization of a safe procedure is caused, in part, by concerns of men and their partners. Some men fear pain and complications; others falsely equate vasectomy with castration or loss of masculinity. It is important to recognize that these misconceptions, concerns, and questions are reflected in the professional community as well. There is little agreement on some of the basic standards regarding vasectomy and its outcomes, follow-up, and complications. For instance, is one method of vasectomy better than others? Which adverse outcomes are considered complications, and which are merely a normal consequence of the procedure? Is there a difference between the outcomes achieved with the various occlusion techniques? What is the recommendation regarding submitting a segment of vas deferens to the pathologist, and what are the legal ramifications of not doing so? How many postvasectomy semen analyses are necessary, and is complete azoospermia required to assure a man of his sterility? As with any surgical procedure, especially those that are elective and have alternatives, the medico-legal issues are significant and are a constant source of concern for the practicing urologist. The first part of this issue addresses these important matters and attempts to provide the practitioner with guidance and answers.

The second half of this issue concentrates on vasectomy reversal. Although, as stated earlier, vasectomy should be considered a permanent procedure, nearly 6% of men who undergo vasectomy ultimately desire a reversal. Divorce and remarriage is the most common reason men seek vasectomy reversals, but many men undergoing reconstruction have the same partner and simply desire more children. There are a variety of personal and social reasons for these decisions. Many individuals regard vasectomy reversal as a new procedure with poor success. Others are under the impression that it is more expensive and less successful than other options. This issue of the *Urology Clinics of North America* provides the reader with the appropriate historical information and discusses the evolution of the technique. As in many surgical procedures, advances have affected success rates significantly. The success rates, as well as the factors predicting success, are reviewed here. Finally, in the era of evidence-based medical decisions, no discussion of vasectomy reversal would be complete if it did not address the cost effectiveness of vasectomy reversal relative to the effective and now well-established alternative of sperm acquisition in conjunction with in vitro fertilization.

Vasectomy continues to be a significant form of contraception. Vasectomy reversal is a consequence of the success of this procedure. We

Urol Clin N Am 36 (2009) xiii–xiv
doi:10.1016/j.ucl.2009.06.001

believe this issue will provide the practitioner with the essential information to guide patients interested in both procedures. The patient will be better informed, and thus the urologist can feel that he or she has fulfilled the obligation to inform the patient fully.

Jay I. Sandlow, MD
Department of Urology
Medical College of Wisconsin
9200 West Wisconsin Avenue
Milwaukee, WI 53226, USA

Harris M. Nagler, MD, FACS
The Albert Einstein College of
Medicine of Yeshiva University
Sol and Margaret Berger Department of Urology
Academic Affairs/Graduate Medical Education
Beth Israel Medical Center
10 Union Square East, Suite 3A
New York, NY 10003, USA

E-mail addresses:
jsandlow@mcw.edu (J.I. Sandlow)
HNagler@chpnet.org (H.M. Nagler)

History of Vasectomy

Yefim R. Sheynkin, MD, FACS

KEYWORDS

• Vasectomy • History • Techniques • Indications

Vasectomy as a medical term is a misnomer because only part of the vas deferens is excised during the procedure. It has been used in the literature to describe a wide range of procedures including partial vasectomy, vasal transection, vasoligation, and vasal occlusion. Vas deferens as an anatomic structure was not a subject of significant clinical and research interest until the nineteenth century. It is difficult, however, to find another surgical procedure as simple as vasectomy that has sparked so much medical and social controversies for more than a century. Vasectomy is a historical, social, philosophic, medical, demographic, and legal phenomenon. It is not surprising that the history of this procedure combines not only a constant quest for ideal technique and better results but also misconceptions, false beliefs, and erroneous indications.

EARLY EXPERIMENTAL AND CLINICAL WORKS ON VASECTOMY

Herophilus (335 BC–280 BC) provided the first account of the testicles, epididymis, vas deferens, seminal vesicles, spermatic artery, and spermatic vein.[1] The vas deferens was first mentioned much later by another ancient physician, Rufus of Ephesus (late first century AD), in one of the first known books on anatomic nomenclature "De nominatione partium hominis" ("On the naming of the parts of the body"), where it was called Πόροί σπερματίκοί.[2] For the following centuries, the amount of neologisms in anatomy was unprecedented because it was necessary to describe and name new things. Thus, vas deferens as a structure in the ancient literature was called "evacuatorium" or "expulsorium seminis," "vas nervosum," "canales" or "pori," even "itinera seminaria" or "venae genitals," all of these being different versions of the Greek translation of "poroi spermatikoi."[3]

Vas deferens (vās, duct + in dēferēns, present participle of dēferre, to carry away) was supposedly named by Mondino dei Liuzzi or Mundinus (1275–1327), anatomist from Bologna.[4,5] His book "De Anatome" (Anothomia) was published in 1316 and widely used in European medical schools for more than 300 years. In the chapter "De anothomia vasorum spermaticorum et testiculorum," he described vasa spermatica praeparantia (semen-preparing vessels that carry semen to the testes) and vasa spermatica deferentia (semen-delivering vessels), that carried semen away from the testes (**Fig. 1**). In his books "Commentary on the Anatomy of Mundinus" (1521) and the famous "Isagogae Brevis" ("A Short Introduction to Anatomy," 1522), another famous Italian anatomist, Berengario da Carpi (1460–1530), mentioned the presence of descending vessels carrying sperm down to the testes and contiguous with them ascending vessels, vasa deferentia (vasa spermatica), which carry sperm away. "Their substance is white and harder than that of the other vessels. These vasa deferentia in the male ascend from the testes to the pubic bone... These vessels bent back within the belly descend between the rectum and the bladder, and there they dilate into many caverns..."[6]

Regnier de Graaf (1641–1673) must be credited for the detailed description and the first experimental work on the vas deferens. In his book "De Vivorum Organis Generationi Inservientibus" (1668), he described vas semen deferens as a "body like large nerve, round white, rather hard and with manifest cavity. So that the cavity may be seen better, a vas deferens should be opened the breadth of 6 or 7 fingers above the testicle and air pumped in the direction of the testicle, or better a coloured liquid injected by means of syringe. The vessel will distend" (**Fig. 2**). In his animal experiments, De Graaf "firmly bound the vas deferens of one testicle in a dog or some other

Department of Urology, Health Science Center, Level 9, Room 040, State University of New York at Stony Brook, Stony Brook, NY 11794-8093, USA
E-mail address: ysheynkin@notes.cc.sunysb.edu

Urol Clin N Am 36 (2009) 285–294
doi:10.1016/j.ucl.2009.05.007

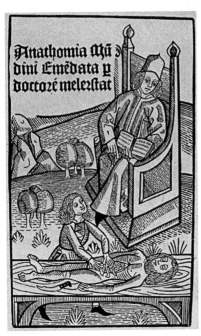

Fig. 1. Mondino dei Liuzzi (1275–1327). Line block after a woodcut, c. 1493. (*Courtesy of* Wellcome Trust, London, UK.)

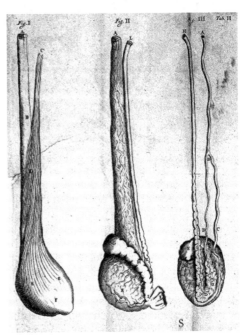

Fig. 2. From Regnier de Graaf "De virorum organis generationi inservientibus, de clysteribus et de usu siphonis in anatomia," 1668. (*Courtesy of* Wellcome Trust, London, UK.)

animal before coitus" and then observed "the tubules of the testicle fill with seminal matter in such way that anyone at all can perceive them.[7]"

John Hunter[8] first described absence of the vas deferens in a cadaver in 1737. More advanced experimental work on the vas deferens was performed by Sir Astley Cooper[9] in the beginning of the nineteenth century. He found that ligation of the dog's vas deferens, unlike ligation of the testicular artery and vein, does not produce a "gangrened and sloughed" testicle. Complete occlusion of the vas deferens caused enlargement of the testis and epididymis, which was also filled with spermatozoa. After 6 years of observation, spermatozoa were found in the epididymis, which confirmed intact sperm production after vasal occlusion.

The effect of vasectomy or vasal occlusion on spermatogenesis was studied later by many researchers with initially controversial reports. Working on dogs and rabbits, Gosselin and Brissaud noted normal spermatogenesis after ligation or resection of the vas deferens.[10–12] Gosselin also dissected human cadavers and observed that entirely blocked vas deferens was associated with an enlarged epididymis that contained quantities of spermatozoa. These observations were confirmed by Curling in 1866.[13] Bouin and Ancel (1903) declared that closing the outlet from the testis invariably leads to degeneration of the germinal tissue, however.[14] This opinion was

supported by works of Tiedje and Sand,[15,16] who also used vasoligation in clinical practice. In 1924, Moore and Quick and then Oslund[17,18] studied the effect of vasectomy on rabbits, rats, and guinea pigs. They concluded that vasectomy alone does not cause degeneration of germ cells. Clinical evidence of preserved spermatogenesis was provided by Posner, who reported that "by puncture of the testis he had withdrawn living spermatozoa 10–17 years after occlusion of the epididymis by gonorrheal invasion." William Belfield, on making an anastomosis of epididymis and vas for cure of sterility, found spermatozoa present 14 years after the occlusion of the epididymis had occurred.[19] By the first quarter of the twentieth century, research and clinical observation revealed no bad effects after vasectomy/vasal occlusion.

VASECTOMY IN CLINICAL PRACTICE: THE BEGINNING

Clinical use of vasectomy can be traced back to the 1880s. Since the first orchiectomy was performed by Louis Auguste Mercier in 1857 for the treatment of enlarged prostate, castration has been used to reduce obstructive symptoms of prostatic hypertrophy and improve micturition.[20] The earliest reference to section of vasa deferentia as an alternative procedure to castration to achieve prostatic atrophy was made by Felix Guyon in 1885 (**Fig. 3**).[21] Five years later, in 1890, James Ewing Mears also suggested vasectomy for the same reasons. Karl Gustav Lennander from Uppsala University (Sweden) advocated vasectomy as a substitute for castration "as a means of relieving ills consecutive to prostatic hypertrophy in 1894.[22] Pavone and Isnardi described prostatic atrophy as a result of vasectomy.[23] Reginald Harrison performed more than 100 vasectomies between 1893 and 1900 (**Fig. 4**). He found that "the usual effect of vasectomy is to induce shrinkage of the hypertrophied prostate" and restore natural micturition. Harrison performed vasectomy by excision of the portion of the vas deferens but later substituted it with torsion of the vas deferens for vasal obliteration "with the pair of Spencer Wells forceps, through a small incision over the duct." In this way, the vas is seized and bared and a small portion of it is torsed out, no ligature being required. A 7- or or 10-day interval in dealing with the two vasa is advised."[24] Harrison was probably the first physician who also noticed reconnection of the divided portion of the vas deferens. "It was found six months after a portion of one of the vasa had been excised and the ends ligatured in a loop that the divided ends had reunited and the continuity and use of the duct has been reestablished."[25] Vasectomy enjoyed popularity for

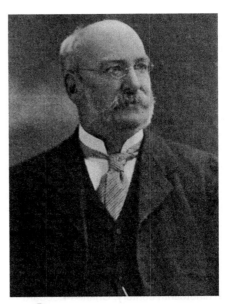

Fig. 4. Reginald Harrison (1837–1908). (*From* Obituary. Reginald Harrison, FRSCEng. BMJ 1908;1(2462):601; with permission.)

a short time because it was considered a method of minimal harm and high efficacy.

Further experience, however, lowered the expectation of micturition improvement after vasectomy. In 1895, Guyon failed to obtain any substantial loss of the bulk of the prostate in four different experiments. Wood[26] reviewed 192 cases of vasectomies and reported improvement in urination in 15%, no changes in 15%, and deaths in 6.7%. Wallace[27] concluded that "a single or double vasectomy is useless as a means of producing prostatic atrophy." Shortly afterwards, this method had lost its recognition as a treatment for prostatic hypertrophy, especially with further developments of surgical treatment of enlarged prostate.

Wood[26] noticed that vasectomy was successfully performed for the relief of painful recurrent orchitis, which "quite justified this operation apart from any intention to affect the prostate." Although prostatectomy has become a more commonly performed procedure, epididymitis was recognized as a far too frequent surgical complication. Vasectomy was recommended for prevention of postoperative epididymitis at the beginning of the twentieth century. In 1904, Robert Proust,[28] a French urologist and brother of famous writer Marcel Proust, mentioned vasectomy at the time of prostatectomy. It was also recommended by Jose Albarran in 1909.[29] Allea described a temporary through-the-skin vasoligation technique.[21]

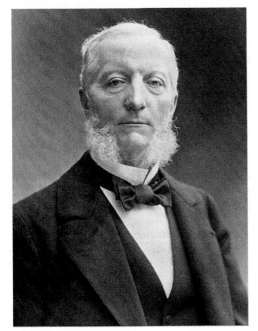

Fig. 3. Felix Guyon (1831–1920). (*Courtesy of* Wellcome Trust, London, UK.)

This technique was discouraged because of difficulties feeling and isolating the vas, however. Meltzer (1928)[30] recommended bilateral vasectomy, rather than vasoligation, as "a definitive prophylactic measure against the painful complication of epididymitis." Scrotal vasectomy had been a popular—albeit controversial—procedure before, during, or after open prostatectomy and even transurethral resection of the prostate (TURP) for almost 80 years. With improved surgical techniques and new effective antibiotics, the incidence of epididymitis diminished drastically. One of the last prospective studies conducted in 1975 showed that vasectomy does not reduce the incidence of epididymitis and its routine use in prostatic surgery is not indicated.[31]

THE FOUNTAIN OF YOUTH

In the nineteenth century, Charles-Edouard Brown Sequard (1817–1894) coined the word "rejuvenation," and the interest of defeating old age flourished in the early twentieth century. After 20 years of sophisticated animal research on testicular function, Eugen Steinach (1861–1944),[32] an Austrian physiologist, professor of biology at the University of Vienna, and director of the city's Biologic Institute of the Academy of Science, published his famous book "Rejuvenation Through the Experimental Revitalization of the Aging Puberty Gland"(1920). He reported degeneration of the germinal epithelium and hypertrophy of the interstitial (Leydig) cells after unilateral vasectomy or vasoligation. This, in turn, stimulates the production of germ cells by the opposite testis and returns old animals to a functional condition. Steinach announced that he had rejuvenated a senile male rat with vasoligation and that the technique can be used on humans. Surgery of the vas deferens (vasectomy or vasoligation) was termed a Steinach I procedure; introduced later was the less popular ligation of the efferent ductules between testis and epididymis, known as a Steinach II operation (**Fig. 5**).

On November 1, 1918, Dr. Robert Lichtenstern performed the Steinach procedure on Anton W., a 43-year-old coachman who suffered from chronic fatigue. "The patient presented with the appearance of an exhausted and prematurely old man," Steinach reported in his book.[32] The procedure resulted in long-lasting improvement. It brought Steinach world fame. In April 1923, the New York Times wrote about the "exodus to Vienna" of doctors who hoped to learn the secret of the Steinach operation.

Thousands of Steinach operations were performed in the United States and around the world. Before his planned visit to America, the New York

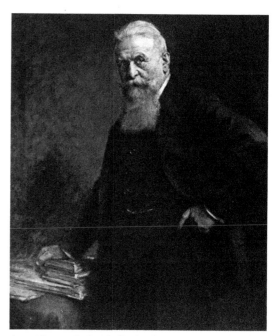

Fig. 5. Eugen Steinach (1861–1944). (Courtesy of Wellcome Trust, London, UK.)

Times wrote: "Dr. Steinach Coming to Make Old Young." He was so famous that his name became a verb: men were "Steinached."[33] Eugen Steinach was nominated unsuccessfully for a Nobel Prize in physiology six times between 1921 and 1938.

On November 17,1923, the Viennese urologist Victor Blum performed a Steinach operation on Sigmund Freud, who "hoped that it might bar the recurrence of his jaw cancer and might even improved his sexuality, general condition and his capacity to work." After the procedure, Freud was ambiguous about its effect. Another famous person, the Nobel Prize winner in literature W.B. Yeats, underwent a vasectomy on April 6, 1934, at the age of 69. "It revived my creative power and…sexual desire," he wrote in 1937.[34]

Medical views on the rejuvenation vasectomy procedure ranged from those of devotees, such as Robert Lichtenstern and Peter Schmidt in Germany, Harry Benjamin in America, and Norman Haire in England, to scoffers such as Morris Fishbein (1889–1976) the editor of JAMA. Fishbein denounced the Steinach procedure as early as 1927 with the lack of scientifically controlled studies.[34] The procedure was in use until the late 1940s, however. Popularity of rejuvenation by vasectomy gradually declined after isolation of testosterone in 1935. In 1951, the most well-known proponent of the Steinach procedure, Norman Haire, accepted that his belief about rejuvenating consequence of vasectomy was faulty.

The Simon Population Trust, a UK voluntary sterilization organization, declared that the Trust did not recommend vasectomy for rejuvenation only in 1969.[35]

VASECTOMY FOR EUGENIC STERILIZATION

Why not ligate the vas deferens to promote Malthusian ideas? This rhetorical question from editorial comments in 1891 defined a new direction in the vasectomy history for the next half-century.[36] In 1897, Van Meter suggested vasectomy for male sterilization to eradicate hereditary disease from the human family. "Furthermore…we can easily have enacted a law that will provide for the sterilization of all criminals; and thus will crime be wiped out, or, at least, greatly lessened."[37] A.J. Ochsner, surgeon in chief of Augustana Hospital and St. Mary's Hospital in Chicago and the future president of American College of Surgeons, reported two vasectomies performed in 1897 to relieve urinary retention secondary to enlarged prostate. The procedure consisted of the resection of the vasa deferentia on both sides through an incision less than 1 in long just below the external inguinal ring. Both patients had no harmful effect or impairment of sexual desire. Ochsner concluded that vasectomy can substitute for castration, which has been recommended as a punishment for certain crimes and had been practiced without legal sanction in many cases. He suggested vasectomy for sterilizing habitual criminals and "chronic inebriates, imbeciles, perverts and paupers" to protect the community at large without harming the criminals.[38] Dr. Daniel Brown of Chicago also recommended vasectomy for eugenic purposes in his address "Medical Aspects of Crime," which was read before the American Medical Association in 1899.[39]

The first eugenic sterilization was performed by Dr. Harry Sharp, chief physician of the Indiana State Reformatory (**Fig. 6**). The inmate named Clawson insisted on castration to stop excessive masturbation. Sharp offered him a vasectomy which he performed on October 12, 1899. A semen sample was examined later under the microscope and "found to be sterile." The inmate reportedly "stopped masturbating, his mind was better." Although the first vasectomies were performed via low inguinal incision, later Sharp used the English method, "which selects the scrotal region as the site of the operation." The vas deferens was clasped between thumb and index finger and severed via the short longitudinal skin incision which was left open at the end of the operation. Both Ochsner and Sharp practiced open-end vasectomy. Dr. Sharp presented his first paper on the subject at the

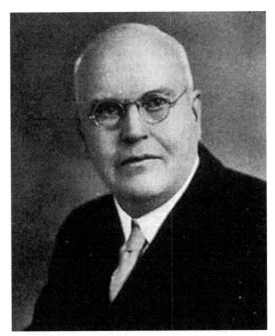

Fig. 6. Harry C. Sharp. (*From* Popenoe P. The progress of eugenic sterilization. J Hered 1934;25:19–26; with permission.)

Mississippi Valley Medical Association meeting at Put-In-Bay in the fall of 1901.[39]

Forty-two similar operations were performed by 1902; 176 were performed by 1907.[40] During the next few years, several articles by physicians claimed that vasectomy offers a solution to the problem of limiting the birth of defective persons. In 1907, the governor of Indiana signed the nation's first sterilization law to initiate the involuntary sterilization of any habitual criminal, rapist, idiot, or imbecile committed to the state institution and diagnosed by physicians as "unimprovable."[41] By 1909, Sharp performed 280 such procedures and quickly emerged as the national authority on eugenic sterilization. He published a pamphlet, "Vasectomy," with an affixed tear-out postcard with a preprinted message supporting sterilization law. In 1910, Sharp demonstrated vasectomy to a doctor from Russia who attended an international conference under the auspices of the American Prison Association.[39] By 1917, 15 of the United States successfully passed laws authorizing vasectomy for various conditions and crimes. By 1937, it had increased to 32 states. The first European Sterilization Law was passed in Switzerland in 1928 followed by Denmark, Germany, Sweden, Norway, and Finland in 1936.[35] The practice of involuntary sterilization gradually ceased and virtually stopped by the 1960s.

POPULATION CONTROL AND FAMILY PLANNING

In 1909, William Belfield, professor of surgery at Rush Medical College, wrote about married men who chose vasectomy rather than criminal abortion to prevent the transmission to offspring of their own hereditary taints, such as insanity and syphilis.[42] Vincent O'Connor[43] summarized the reasons for surgical sterilization of men: (1) prevention of the insane, the criminal, or the perverse from producing offspring, (2) precarious health of the wife, which increased the risk of bearing children, and the wife being unable or refusing to undergo tubal ligation, (3) agreement between husband and wife to prevent pregnancy, (4) prevention of the occurrence of epididymitis, a routine procedure in many clinics in the treatment of prostatism, (5) rejuvenation (Steinach), a false physiologic assumption and clinical failure, and (6) mass sterilization for the purpose of racial limitation, as evidenced by recent Nazi treatment of persons of Jewish, Polish, and other nationalities. It was the first time voluntary vasectomy was clearly mentioned for family planning. Vasectomy for voluntary sterilization was not widely performed, however. "The person who seeks to have himself sterilized…does it so secretly and for what he considers strong personal reasons. The patient frequently encounters difficulty in persuading a competent surgeon to perform this procedure because in most states there is question as to its legality and the surgeon exposed himself to a possible suit for malpractice."[43] In 1953, the British Family Planning Association recommended that couples who request sterilization on the ground that it is easier and more reliable than birth control should receive a lesson in social responsibility.[44] Before 1969, the American College of Obstetricians and Gynecologists recommended restricting voluntary sterilization to men or women whose age multiplied by number of children equaled or exceeded 120.

Although vasectomy as a contraceptive procedure for family planning was not commonly used in the developed countries, the procedure was successfully introduced to control rapidly growing population in certain developing Asian countries. India launched a massive program and became the first country in the world to make it an official government policy in 1952.[45] The approaches to encourage men to be sterilized included outreach to men at workplaces or in rural communities using mobile units, vasectomy "camps" and "festivals," special clinic hours, and settings that were considered more appealing to men. In India, the Ernakulam camps achieved 78,000 male sterilizations annually, whereas in Gujarat camps sterilization was performed on more than 200,000 men in 2 months.[46] In Thailand, large numbers of men receive vasectomies during special festivals held on the King's birthday.[47] Quality of care has been a problem in many of the mass camps.

One of the most important and controversial elements of vasectomy promotion in Asia historically has been incentive payments to providers and acceptors, however. In some countries, major incentive payments were used that bordered on coercion because the money offered for sterilization equaled or surpassed monthly salaries. These aggressive programs were focused on mostly poor and less informed social groups. This approach to vasectomy reached a new level during India's Emergency period (1975–1977). Over these 2 years, during which the government made an extraordinary effort toward the goal of reducing the population, almost 7% of all Indian couples were sterilized.[44] A total of 6.2 million vasectomies were performed in 1976, almost 5 million more than in 1975.[48] This task was accomplished through undeniably coercive means. In some Indian states, police, school teachers, and other government employees participated in recruiting men to have vasectomy. When the Emergency ended in 1977, the government was preparing laws to make small families compulsory. Reaction against the coercive vasectomy program and population control helped bring down the Gandhi government in March 1977.[49]

In the ensuing years, the entire family planning program was toned down, and vasectomy in particular "lost its credibility and never regained its popularity." Vasectomy, the dominant family planning method in India for 20 years, was almost entirely replaced by female sterilization.[49] Ironically, the worldwide discussion about the importance of male participation in family planning had started after the decline in vasectomy programs. The First International Conference on Vasectomy was conducted in October 1982 in Colombo, Sri Lanka. Seventy leading professionals from 25 countries reviewed vasectomy efforts, examined the main barriers to accessibility, and reported ways to overcome these barriers.[50]

In the United States, the Association for Voluntary Sterilization promoted the benefits of voluntary sterilization as a means of family planning. Its predecessor, the Sterilization League of New Jersey, was formed in 1937 to support the eugenic sterilization of the physically and developmentally disabled and persons with mental illness. Between 1943 and 1964, the organization changed its name several times. It was known successively as Birthright (1943–1950), the Human Betterment Association of America (1950–1962), and the Human

Betterment Association for Voluntary Sterilization (1962–1964) before becoming the Association for Voluntary Sterilization in 1965. The Association for Voluntary Sterilization changed its name to the Association for Voluntary Surgical Contraception during the 1980s, was renamed the Association for Voluntary Surgical Contraception International in 1994, and became Engender Health in 2001.[51]

The data on vasectomy as a contraceptive method in the 1950s are limited. In California, Poffenberger published his report on 2000 voluntary vasectomies performed between 1956 and 1961. He reported that "not only were men pleased with the result of the operation but they talked about its advantages freely and attempted, often with success, to convince others to have it done. In some cases, men came several hundred miles to have the operation. Of the total sample, only 14.5% reported one or more physical reasons motivating them to seek a vasectomy. The rest gave no medical reason for desiring the operation."[52] The largest single objection for performing voluntary elective vasectomy was a legal one from a misunderstanding of the law. In 1963, the American Medical Association legal counsel advised that "outside of the two states where nontherapeutic sterilization is expressly prohibited by law (Connecticut and Utah), the physician who performs these procedures does not expose himself unduly to civil or criminal liability."[53] Between 1963 and 1967, already 40,000 vasectomies had been performed annually in the United States.[54] By 1991, the number of vasectomies performed annually increased to 493,487 and reached 526,501 in 2002 (approximately 10/1000 men aged 25–49 years).[55,56]

Vasectomy use worldwide is different from country to country. Marie Stopes International family planning services in the United Kingdom has advertised contraceptive vasectomy since 1958.[57] In the 1970s and 1980s, new statutory provisions in several Western European countries made voluntary sterilization legal. In England and Wales, vasectomy was incorporated into the National Health Service in 1972. A short time later, Scandinavian statutes introduced the right to obtain voluntary sterilization upon request for all men over 25 years of age in Denmark, Sweden, Norway, and Iceland. The lower limit of 25 was also enacted in Austria. In 1978, Italy legalized voluntary sterilization; in that year the operation became legal, by implication, in Luxembourg. In 1983, Spain and Turkey repealed their antisterilization laws. In 1975, the high degree of consensus of European countries on full liberalization of voluntary sterilization was expressed by an international

act. The Council of Ministers of the Council of Europe unanimously voted in Resolution No. 75 on November 14, 1975.[29] By this resolution, the Committee recommended the 21 member countries to "make sterilization (for family planning purposes) available as a medical service."[58] In France, vasectomy was considered an illicit procedure under the nineteenth century "Napoleon code," which proscribed acts of so called "self mutilation." The birth control charity Marie Stopes International even offered a "vasectomy tourist service "to the United Kingdom on its Web site.[59] The procedure became legal in France in 2001.

Although data on vasectomy worldwide are incomplete, the countries with the highest prevalence of this sterilization method are New Zealand, United Kingdom, Canada, United States, South Korea, Australia, Switzerland, China, and Denmark.

TECHNICAL EVOLUTION OF VASECTOMY

From the early days of vasectomy use in clinical practice, surgeons throughout the world have tried to find a better way to perform this procedure. The driving forces behind the multiple modifications of vasectomy were simplification and shortening the procedure, concerns over the recanalization, and, later, possibility of vasectomy reversal. More than 30 different techniques of surgical approach, section, and occlusion of the vas deferens have been described in the literature.[60]

Early vasectomies were performed via an inguinal approach. One of the first modifications, the "English method," selects the scrotal region as the site of the operation.[24] Harrison excised the portion of the vas deferens via two incisions over the vas on each side of the scrotum and ligated the ends in a loop.[25] Alternatively, a loop of the vas was gently drawn out through the wound with a blunt hook. "The loop is then encircled below the hook with a silk ligature…which is tightly knotted. The …extraneous portion of the vas removed with scissors and the pedicle dropped into its place."[61] Van Meter in 1897 and Sharp 1909 recommended an open-end procedure with ligation of the abdominal end and leaving open the testicular end "in order that the secretion of the testicle may be emptied around the vessels of pampiniform plexus and there be absorbed."[37,40]

In 1955, Jhaver introduced the single incision approach for bilateral vasectomy. After performing a large series of vasectomy operations by this method, he published this technique in 1958.[62,63] This approach was later questioned by Schmidt, who thought it could lead to operating twice on the same vas deferens, missing the other completely.

The possibility of spontaneous vasal reanastomosis, which was clinically observed by Harrison in 1900, was confirmed by Rolnick,[64] who reported in 1924 that the canine vas can regenerate over long distances by endothelialization of its sheath. Since then, many methods of the occlusion of the vasal ends have been introduced to avoid recanalization. Besides ligation of the cut vasal ends, Strode (1937) first attempted a fascial interposition between the ligated end of the vas deferens. He buried the proximal (testicular) end within the surrounding fascia distal (abdominal) end outside the fascia.[65] In 1966, Schmidt introduced fulguration of the vasal lumen with electrocautery and later with red-hot wire cautery to effectively and quickly seal the vas deferens without additional occlusion and removal of portion of the vas. He also closed the vasal sheath over the distal cut end to prevent recanalization.[66,67]

Jhaver[68] started to use one tantalum medium clip instead of ligatures on each divided vasal end, whereas Moss[69] advocated two tantalum clips across each divided end for occlusion. The vasectomy failure rate was 1.2% with one clip and 0% with two clips. Craft[70] suggested irrigation of the distal cut end of the vas with sterile water to facilitate azoospermia.

By 1972, the surgical modifications seemed to have been exhausted. In 1973, the no-scalpel vasectomy technique was developed by Dr. Shunqiang Li and associates.[71] The procedure was done without a skin incision using two instruments: a ring forceps to hold the vas deferens without piercing the skin (similar to vas clamp designed by Allea in 1928) and a sharp hemostat. Since then, no-scalpel vasectomy has been widely promulgated and practiced in China as a routine sterilization method, with 8 million no-scalpel vasectomy procedures performed on Chinese men between 1974 and 1988. In June 1985, an expert group of physicians sponsored by the Association for Voluntary Surgical Contraception visited the Chongqing Family Planning Scientific Research Institute in China to learn the new vasectomy technique.[72,73] The first no-scalpel vasectomy performed in the United States was by Dr. Mark Goldstein, who was a member of that international team, at the New York Hospital– Cornell Medical Center in 1985. In November 1986, the 1st International Training Course on no-scalpel vasectomy was conducted in Bangkok, Thailand.[72] The no-scalpel vasectomy technique has rapidly gained popularity among surgeons and patients because of shorter operative time,

less tissue injury, less postoperative swelling and pain, and a lower complication rate.

Vasal occlusion without division of the vas deferens has been an attractive concept for many years because of its simplicity. Allea recommended temporary percutaneous ligation of the vas deferens with silk ligature before prostate surgery to prevent epididymitis. The ligature was removed in 15 days. Microscopic studies in four patients revealed complete obstruction of the vas after removal of the ligature.[21] The idea of reversible vasal occlusion was popular in the 1960s. Procedures using the new techniques of vasal occlusion, including a "plug" of plastic materials, the intravas device, vas clip, and vas valve, have been attempted.[74] In 2002, the VasClip, a small implantable biocompatible lock made of a medical-grade polymer, was approved by the US Food and Drug Administration in 2002 with an indication for ligation of the vas deferens. The VasClip was found to fail at an unexpectedly high rate and has since been taken off the market, however.[75]

Recently the feasibility of thermal occlusion of the vas deferens with noninvasive, transcutaneous high intensity focused ultrasound has been demonstrated on animal models.[76] After more than a century of controversies, improvements and technical innovations, modern vasectomy has become a safe, effective, and permanent male contraceptive procedure. However, the ideal technique has yet to be found. Predictably, minimally invasive methods of permanent vasal occlusion will continue to evolve.

REFERENCES

1. Libby W. The history of medicine in its salient features. Boston (MA): Houghton Mifflin Company; 1922. p. 50–1.
2. Rufus of Ephesus. Names of the parts of the body. In: Daremberg C, Ruelle CE, editors. Oeuvres de Rufus d'Ephese [transl]. Amsterdam: Adolf M.Hakkert; 1963. p. 67–8. (reprint of the Paris, J.B Bailliere, 1879 edition).
3. Ivanova A, Holomanova A. The anatomic nomenclature by Vesalius. Bratisl Lek Listy 2001;102(3): 169–73.
4. The American heritage dictionary of the English language. 4th edition. Houghton Mifflin Harcourt; 2000.
5. Bresadola M, Fezzi P. Mondino dei Liuzzi: Anothomia a cura di Piero Giorgi. International Centre for the History of Universities and Science. Available at: http://cis.alma.unibo.it/Mondino/auctor.htm. Accessed June 2, 2009. [Latin].
6. da Carpi JB. A short introduction to anatomy (Isagogae Breves). Translated by L.R. Lind, with

Anatomical Notes by Paul G. Roofe. Chicago: University of Chicago Press; 1959 [Latin].

7. Jocelyn HD, Setchell BP. Regnier de Graaf on the human reproductive organs: an annotated translation of Tractatus de Virorum Organis Generationi Inservientibus (1668) and De Mulierub Organis Generationi Inservientibus Tractatus Novus (1672). J Reprod Fertil Suppl 1972;17:1–76 [Latin].

8. Hunter J. Observation on the glands situated between the rectum and bladder, called vesiculae seminales. In: Palmer JF, editor. Complete Works. London: Longman, Reese, Orm, Brown, Green & Longman; 1737. p. 20–34.

9. Cooper A. Observation on the structure and diseases of the testis. London: Longman; 1830.

10. Jhaver PS, Ohri BB. The history of experimental and clinical work on vasectomy. J Int Coll Surg 1960;33: 482–6.

11. Gosselin P. Nouvelles etudes sur l'obliteration des voies spermatique et sur sterilite consecutive a l'epididymite bilaterale. Arch Gen de Med 1847; Serie 5, vol II, p. 257–70 [French].

12. Brissaud E. Les effects de la ligature du canal deferent. Arch D Physiol 1880;S2:769–89 [French].

13. Curling TB. A practical treatise on diseases of the testis and of the spermatic cord and scrotum, 2nd edition. Philadelphia: Blanchard and Lea; 1856.

14. Bouin F, Ancel P. Recheres sur les cellules interstitielles du testicule des mammiferes. Arch d Zool Exper 1903;S4(1):437–523 [French].

15. Tiedje P. Changes in testes after ligation. Deutsch med Wchnschr 1921;47:352–63 [German].

16. Sand K. Experiences sur la resection du vas deferens. J dePhysiol et de Path Gen 1921;19:494–503 [French].

17. Oslund R. Vasectomy on rats and guinea pigs. Am J Physiol 1924;67:422–43.

18. Moore CR, Quick WMJ. Vasectomy in rabbits. Am J Anat 1924;34:317–36.

19. After-effects of vasectomy. [editorial comments]. JAMA 1909;24:1348.

20. Ricketts BM. Surgery of the prostate, pancreas, diaphragm, spleen, thyroid and hydrocephalus: a historical review. Cincinnati: Lancet Clin; 1904.

21. Alyea EP. Vaso-ligation: a preventive of epididymitis before and after prostatectomy. J Urol 1928;19:65–80.

22. Gallant AE. Sterilization of the unfit by vasectomy. Med Times 1915;43:39.

23. Harrison R. Diseases of genito-urinary system: the year-book for treatment for physicians. Philadelphia: Cassell and Company Limited; 1896. p. 267.

24. Harrison R. Remarks on vasectomy relative to enlarged prostate and bladder atony. Lancet 1900; 155:1275–6.

25. Harrison R. Illustration of vasectomy or obliteration of the seminal ducts relative to hypertrophy of the prostate and bladder atony. Lancet 1900;156:96–7.

26. Wood AC. The results of castration and vasectomy in hypertrophy of prostate gland. Ann Surg 1900; 32:309–50.

27. Wallace CS. The results of castration and vasectomy upon the prostate gland in the enlarged and normal condition. Trans Path Soc Lond 1905;56:80–106.

28. Proust R. La prostatectomie dans l'hypertrophie de la prostate. Paris: Mason et Cie; 1904 [French].

29. Albarran J. Medicine operatoire de voies urinaires. Paris: 1909 [French].

30. Meltzer M. Bilateral vasectomy for prevention of epididymitis in prostatism. NY State J Med 1928; 28:1290–2.

31. Wagenaar J. Vasectomy in prostatic surgery. Eur Urol 1975;1(6):275–7.

32. Steinach Eugen. Verjüngung durch experimentelle neubelebung der alternden pubertätsdrüse. [Rejuvenation by experimental revitalization of the ageing puberty gland]. Archiv für Entwicklungsmechanik der Organismen 1920;46:557–610 [German].

33. Sengoopta C. Tales from the Vienna labs: the Eugen Steinach–Harry Benjamin correspondence. Newsletter of the rare book room. New York: The New York Academy of Medicine; 2000;2:5–7.

34. Wyndham D. Versemaking and lovemaking: W.B. Yeats "strange second puberty." Norman Haire and Steinach rejuvenation operation. J Hist Behav Sci 2003;39:25–50.

35. Wolfers D, Wolfers H. Vasectomania. Fam Plann Perspect 1973;5:196–9.

36. Why not ligate the vas deferens? Med Rec 1891;39: 266.

37. Van Meter ME. Some new methods in surgery. Transaction of the National Eclectic Medical Association 1898;25:69–75.

38. Ochsner AJ. Surgical treatment of habitual criminals. JAMA 1899;32:867–8.

39. Kantor WM. Beginning of sterilization in America. J Hered 1937;28:374–6.

40. Sharp HC. Vasectomy as a means of preventing procreation in defectives. JAMA 1909;53:1897–902.

41. Reilly P. Involuntary sterilization in the United States: a surgical solution. Q Rev Biol 1987;62:153–70.

42. Gallant AE. Sterilization of the unfit by vasectomy. Med Times 1915;43:38–40.

43. O'Connor VJ. Anastomosis of vas deferens after purposeful division for sterility. JAMA 1948;3: 162–3.

44. Stallworthy J, Walker K, Malleson J, et al. Problems of fertility in general practice. London: Cassell and Co; 1953.

45. Kashyap KN. Effects of vasectomy on population control and problems of reanastomosis. Proc R Soc Med 1973;66:51–2.

46. Ross JA, Hong S, Huber D. Voluntary sterilization: an international fact book association for voluntary sterilization. New York, 1985.

47. Nirapathpongporn A, Huber DH, Krieger JN. No-scalpel vasectomy at the King's birthday vasectomy festival. Lancet 1990;335(8694):894–5.

48. Liskin L, Pile JM, Quillin WF. Vasectomy: safe and simple. Population Reports Series D 1983;4:61–100.

49. Srinivasan K. Regulating reproduction in India's population: efforts, results and recommendations. New Delhi: Sage Publications; 1995.

50. Atkins BS, Jezowski TW. Report on the first international conference on vasectomy. Stud Fam Plann 1983;14:89–95.

51. Blouin F, Jessee WS. The Association for Voluntary Sterilization Records, 1929–1981. Minneapolis: Social Welfare History Archives, University of Minnesota Libraries. Available at: http://special.lib.umn.edu. Accessed June 3, 2009.

52. Poffenberger T. Two thousand voluntary sterilizations performed in California: background factors and comments. Marriage Fam Living 1963;25:469–74.

53. Landis J. Attitudes of individual California physicians and policies of state medical societies on vasectomy for birth control. J Marriage Fam 1966;28:277–83.

54. Davis JE, Hulka JF. Elective vasectomy by American urologists in 1967. Fertil Steril 1970;21:615–21.

55. Mangani R, Haws J, Morgan G. Vasectomy in the United States, 1991 and 1995. Am J Public Health 1999;89:92–4.

56. Barone MA, Hutchinson PL, Johnson CH, et al. Vasectomy in the United States, 2002. J Urol 2006;176:232–6.

57. Vasectomy: follow-up of thousand vasectomies. Cambridge: The Simon Population Trust; 1969.

58. Stepan J. Sterilization: the quiet revolution. People 1985;12(4):30–1.

59. Mayor S. French men invited to become "vasectomy tourists." BMJ 2000;321:470.

60. Klapproth HJ, Young IS. Vasectomy, vas ligation and vas occlusion. Urology 1973;1:292–300.

61. Division of the vas deferens in prostatic hypertrophy. Med Rec 1896;49:696–7.

62. Jhaver PS. Vasectomy after effects, modern techniques, complications, repair. Indian J Med Sci 1973;27:411–6.

63. Ohri BB, Jhaver PS. Single incision single stitch technique for vasectomy. Indian J Surg 1968;20:480–4.

64. Rolnick HC. Regeneration of the vas deferens. Arch Surg 1924;9:188–203.

65. Strode JE. A technique of vasectomy for sterilization. J Urol 1937;37:733–6.

66. Schmidt SS. Prevention of failure in vasectomy. J Urol 1973;109:296–7.

67. Schmidt SS. Techniques and complications of elective vasectomy: the role of spermatic granuloma in spontaneous recanalization. Fertil Steril 1966;17:467–82.

68. Jhaver PS, Davis JE, Lee H, et al. Reversibility of sterilization produced by vas-occlusion clip. Fertil Steril 1971;22:263–9.

69. Moss WM. A sutureless technique for bilateral partial vasectomy. Fertil Steril 1972;23:33–7.

70. Craft I, MCQueen J. Effect of irrigation of the vas on post-vasectomy semen counts. Lancet 1972;1:515–6.

71. Cutting out the scalpel: a unique approach to vasectomies. Interview with Dr. Li Shunqiang, the originator of no-scalpel vasectomy. China Popul Today 1995;12(5–6):25–7.

72. Bing XU, Huang WD. No-scalpel vasectomy outside China. Asian J Androl 2000;2:21–4.

73. Huber D. No-scalpel vasectomy: the transfer of a refined surgical technique from China to other countries. Adv Contracept 1989;5:217–8.

74. Hulka JF, Davis JE. Vasectomy and reversible vaso-occlusion. Fertil Steril 1972;23:683–96.

75. Levine L, Abern M, Lux M. Persistent motile sperm after ligation band vasectomy. J Urol 2006;176:2146–8.

76. Roberts WW, Chan DY, Fried NM, et al. High intensity focused ultrasound ablation of the vas deferens in canine model. J Urol 2002;167:2613–7.

Demographics of Vasectomy—USA and International

John M. Pile, MPH*, Mark A. Barone, DVM, MS

KEYWORDS

- Vasectomy • Prevalence • USA
- Canada • Developing countries

Vasectomy is safer, simpler, less expensive, and equally as effective as female sterilization—yet it remains one of the least known and least used methods of contraception. Worldwide, an estimated 33 million of married women aged 15 to 49 (less than 3%) rely on their partner's vasectomy for contraception (**Table 1**).[1,2]

Female sterilization is approximately twice as common as vasectomy in the developed world, 8 times more common in Asia, and 15 times more common in Latin America and the Caribbean. The gap is likely greater in sub-Saharan Africa; however, rates are too low for accurate comparison. Vasectomy is more common than female sterilization in only five countries—Bhutan, Canada, the Netherlands, New Zealand, and the Great Britain. In Bhutan, vasectomy is 8 times more common than female sterilization; in Great Britain, nearly 3 times as common; in Canada and the Netherlands, twice as common; and in New Zealand, approximately one third more common.[1,2]

The use of vasectomy in the world varies significantly by region and country. In developed countries overall, fewer than 5% of couples rely on vasectomy. In developing countries, the overall prevalence of vasectomy is 2.5%. Prevalence exceeds 10% in eight countries—Australia, Bhutan, Canada, the Netherlands, New Zealand, the Republic of Korea, Great Britain, and the United States (**Table 2**).[1,2] Bhutan has approximately 40% of contracepting couples relying on vasectomy, the highest proportion in the world, followed by New Zealand with approximately 25%, then Canada, the United Kingdom, and the United States at approximately 20% each, and Australia and the Republic of Korea with 12.5% each.

Asia, with a prevalence of 3%, accounts for approximately three fourths of the 32 million couples worldwide who use vasectomy—China and India alone account for 20 million users. In Latin America and the Caribbean the prevalence of vasectomy is only 2%. Puerto Rico has the highest rate in the region, 5.3%. In sub-Saharan Africa less than one tenth of 1% of married women rely on a partner's vasectomy for contraception.

TRENDS IN VASECTOMY PREVALENCE

Globally, after steadily increasing in the 1990s, the number of couples relying on vasectomy has dropped back to a level seen in the early 1980s (**Fig. 1**). In 1982, an estimated 33 million couples were protected from unintended pregnancy by vasectomy.[8] Over the next decade, the number of couples relying on vasectomy increased by approximately 10 million, and in 1991, vasectomy protected approximately 42 million couples from unintended pregnancy.[9] By 2001, however, the number of couples protected by vasectomy had increased by only 1 million, to an estimated 43 million couples.[10] By comparison, the number of couples relying on female sterilization rose from approximately 140 million in 1991 to more than 210 million in 2001.[11] By 2005, the number of vasectomy users had declined slightly to 38 million whereas the number of female sterilizations had risen to 225 million.[12] The most recent estimate (from 2007) suggests that the number of

Programs Division, EngenderHealth, 440 Ninth Avenue, New York, NY 10001, USA
* Corresponding author.
E-mail address: jpile@engenderhealth.org (J.M. Pile).

Urol Clin N Am 36 (2009) 295–305
doi:10.1016/j.ucl.2009.05.006

Table 1
Worldwide use of vasectomy among married women of reproductive age (15–49), 2007

Region	Percent Married Women of Reproductive Age Using	No. of Users (Million)
Africa	~0.1	0.2
Asia	3	22.5
Latin America/Caribbean	2	1.9
Europe	3	2.9
North America	12	4.1
Oceania	10	0.5
World	2.9	32.8

Data from United Nations. World contraceptive use 2007 (wall chart). New York: United Nations, Department of Economic and Social Affairs, Population Division; 2008; and Population Reference Bureau. Family planning worldwide 2008 data sheet. Washington, DC: Population Reference Bureau; 2008.

vasectomy users has dropped to 33 million whereas the number of female sterilization users has remained constant at 225 million.[1,2] Global estimates of contraceptive use are based on national surveys of women of reproductive age, typically aged 15 to 49. Estimates of the prevalence of vasectomy have declined over the past few years as older age cohorts (married women 35 and older) that were more likely to rely on vasectomy have "aged out" of their reproductive years and much larger younger age cohorts (<15) have "aged in." As a result, although overall

Table 2
Countries with highest vasectomy prevalence among married women of reproductive age (15–49) by region and year of survey (1991–2008)

North America/ Europe/Oceania		Asia		Americas		Africa	
New Zealand (1995)	19.3	Bhutan (2000)	13.6	Puerto Rico (2002)	5.3	Namibia (2000)	0.8
Great Britain (2007/08)	16.0	Republic of Korea (1997)	12.7	Brazil (1996)	2.6	South Africa (2003)	0.7
Canada (1995)	15.2	China (2004)	6.7	Mexico (2003)	1.9	Botswana (2000)	0.2
United States (2002)	12.8	Nepal (2006)	5.0	Colombia (2004/05)	1.8	Swaziland (2006/2007)	0.2
Netherlands (1993)	10.5	Iran (2000)	2.8	Guatemala (2002)	1.0	Central African Republic (2006)	0.1
Australia (2008)	11.2	Sri Lanka (2000)	2.1	Nicaragua (2001)	0.5	Democratic Republic Congo (2001)	0.1
Spain (1999)	9.0	Myanmar (2001)	1.5	Haiti (2000)	0.4	Mauritius (2002)	0.1
Switzerland (1994/1995)	8.3	India (2005/2006)	1.0	Peru (2004/2006)	0.4	Rwanda (2007/2008)	0.1
Belgium (1991)	7.0	Thailand (2005/2006)	1.0	Uruguay (2004)	0.4	Sao Tome and Principe (2000)	0.1
Czech Republic (1997)	5.1	Bangladesh (2006)	0.6	Honduras (2005/2006)	0.3	Uganda (2006)	0.1

Data from Refs.[1–7]

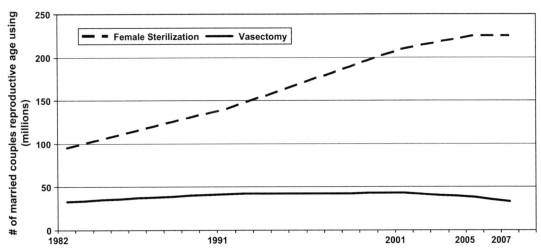

Fig. 1. Estimated number of couples relying on vasectomy worldwide (in millions), 1982–2007. (*Data from* Refs.[1,8–11].)

vasectomy prevalence seems to have declined, in many countries the actual incidence number of procedures performed annually is increasing.

Vasectomy in the United States, Canada, and Other Developed Countries

There is no nationwide surveillance or reporting in place for systematically gathering information on vasectomy incidence or prevalence in the United States. Rather, this information must come from periodic survey or specific research studies. After increasing steadily during the 1960s and 1970s, the rate of vasectomy in the United States leveled off during the 1980s and has remained stable ever since.[13,14] In 1991 and 1995, approximately 500,000 vasectomies were performed in the United States.[15] Although the estimated number performed in 2002, the most recent year for which data are available, was slightly higher at 526,501, the incidence rate has remained unchanged between 1991 and 2002 at approximately 10 per

1000 men aged 25 to 49 (**Fig. 2**).[16] These findings are consistent with results from the National Survey of Family Growth (NSFG)—a periodic survey conducted by the National Center for Health Statistics—indicating that the proportion of women reporting their partner had a vasectomy has remained relatively constant since the late 1980s.[16,17]

In 2002 (the most recent cycle of the NSFG), vasectomy was reported as the fourth most commonly used method (after oral contraceptives, tubal sterilization, and condoms) among women in the United States aged 15 to 44— 5.7% reported they relied on their partner's vasectomy for contraception.[18] For the first time, in 2002, the NSFG included interviews with men aged 15 to 44; 6.2% reported having had a vasectomy.[19] There were wide variations in men's reported use of vasectomy by age, rising from 1.6% to 9.3% from ages 25 to 39 and then increasing dramatically to 18.8% among men 40 to 44 years old.[18]

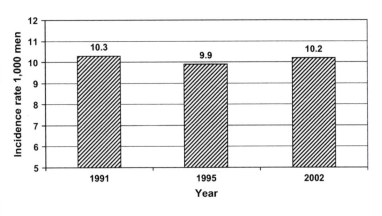

Fig. 2. Vasectomy incidence among men aged 25 to 49 in the United States, 1991 to 2002. (*Data from* Magnani RJ, Haws JM, Morgan GT, et al. Vasectomy in the United States, 1991 and 1995. Am J Public Health 1999; 89[1]:92–4; and Barone MA, Hutchinson PL, Johnson CH, et al. Vasectomy in the United States, 2002. J Urol 2006; 176[1]:232–6.)

There is a large gap in sterilization use between women and men in the United States, with 3 times as many women sterilized than men.[18] Although 16.7 % of women 15 to 44 years old reported female sterilization as their current contraceptive, only 5.7% reported male sterilization.[18] Although the difference decreases among married couples, there are still more than 1.5 times as many couples using female sterilization compared to vasectomy (21.3% versus 12.8%, respectively).[18] There is a wide range of vasectomy prevalence among individual states, ranging from a prevalence of less than 5% in Hawaii, New Jersey, and the District of Columbia to a prevalence of greater than 17% in Idaho, Oregon, Washington, and Vermont (**Table 3**).[20]

Unlike the United States, Canada provides universal health care, and vasectomy is provided to men free of charge through the national health insurance program. It is, therefore, possible to estimate the number of vasectomies performed in Canada using fee-for-service utilization data from the Canadian National Physician Database. According to the most recent report, during 2005 to 2006, approximately 60,908 vasectomies were done in Canada.[20] Using data from the 2006 Canadian census, this translates approximately to a rate of 11 per 1000 men aged 25 to 49.[21] The sterilization usage patterns in Canada show a pattern opposite to that seen in the United States, with more than twice as many men vasectomized than women having had a tubal sterilization in 2005 to 2006 (approximately 60,908 vasectomies versus 27,309 tubal sterilizations).[20]

In Great Britain, the Office for National Statistics conducts annual surveys on contraceptive use among women aged 16 to 49 and men aged 16 to 69. In 2007 to 2008, 16% of all men under 70 years old reported they had a vasectomy and 13% of women reported their partner was sterilized. Among married women, 19% stated their husband had had a vasectomy.[7] Thirty percent of men over age 50 who were interviewed reported having had a vasectomy. The procedure is available free of charge through the National Health Service. The percentage of vasectomies performed by the National Health Service has increased significantly in the past decade, rising from 66% in 20001 to 2002 to 74% in 2007 to 2008.[7]

Table 3
Vasectomy prevalence in the United States and Territories, by state (2002).

<5		5 to <10		10 to <15		15+	
Hawaii	4.9	Illinois	9.8	Wisconsin	14.9	Idaho	19.9
New Jersey	4.7	Virginia	9.3	Wyoming	14.5	Washington	18.5
Guam	3.9	Maryland	9.2	Colorado	14.4	Vermont	17.5
U.S. Virgin Islands	2.1	California	8.8	Maine	14.3	Oregon	17.2
District of Columbia	1.5	Delaware	8.7	Indiana	14.2	Minnesota	16.8
—	—	West Virginia	8.2	North Dakota	14.2	Montana	16.8
—	—	Tennessee	8.1	Alaska	13.8	New Hampshire	16.1
—	—	Nevada	8.1	Ohio	13.7	Michigan	15.7
—	—	Georgia	7.9	Nebraska	13.3	Iowa	15.0
—	—	Massachusetts	7.9	Kansas	13.0	—	—
—	—	North Carolina	7.2	Arkansas	12.5	—	—
—	—	Alabama	7.0	Oklahoma	12.4	—	—
—	—	Kentucky	7.0	South Dakota	11.7	—	—
—	—	New York	6.9	Arizona	11.5	—	—
—	—	South Carolina	6.9	Missouri	11.2	—	—
—	—	Florida	6.8	Utah	10.9	—	—
—	—	Louisiana	6.7	New Mexico	10.4	—	—
—	—	Texas	6.6	Rhode Island	10.2	—	—
—	—	Mississippi	5.8	Connecticut	10.1	—	—
—	—	Puerto Rico	5.4	Pennsylvania	10.1	—	—

Data from Bensyl D, Iuliano D, Carter M, et al. Contraceptive use—United States and territories, Behavioral Risk Factor Surveillance System, 2002. MMWR Surveill Summ 2005;54(6):1–72.

New Zealand has the highest vasectomy prevalence in the world, 19.3%. Widely used since the 1970s, its prevalence surpassed that of female sterilization in the mid-1980s. In the late 1990s a telephone survey found that more than half (57%) of men aged 40 to 49 had had vasectomies.[22] The procedure is popular among all socioeconomic groups. In Australia, vasectomy has increased steadily in popularity since the early 1970s when the Australian Medical Association dropped its opposition to the method.[23]

Vasectomy in Latin America and the Caribbean

Vasectomy use in Latin America and the Caribbean has increased 60-fold in the past 25 years, fourfold in the past 15 years. In 1983, only 30,000 couples were using vasectomy in the region.[8] By 1991, that number had increased to 400,000.[9] In 2007, an estimated 1.9 million couples of reproductive age relied on vasectomy.[2] Nevertheless, the prevalence remains less than 1% in much of the region, the exceptions being Brazil, Colombia, Guatemala, and Mexico, countries that had programs that benefited from significant donor support for vasectomy services in the 1980s and early 1990s (**Fig. 3**).

Vasectomy in Asia

In Asia, vasectomy played a dominant role in the early years of many national family planning programs. In the 1960s and 1970s vasectomy was heavily promoted in Bangladesh, India, Nepal, and the Republic of Korea, and it was not until the late 1970s that female sterilization began to outpace vasectomy.[10] In Nepal, as alternative methods have become available over the past 30 years, vasectomy's percentage of overall contraceptive prevalence has declined from 66% in 1976 to 11% in 2006 (**Fig. 4**).

In India, the high-pressured approach, which included aggressively promoting vasectomy through camps, cash incentives, and reportedly coercive practices, contributed to bringing down the Gandhi government in 1977.[10] Within India today, vasectomy prevalence varies greatly from one state to another, ranging from a high of 6.3% in Himachal Pradesh to a low of less than 0.05% in Mizoram and Nagaland (**Fig. 5**). The government of India recently renewed its attention to vasectomy, and the number of procedures performed in the public sector nearly doubled between 2006 to 2007 and 2007 to 2008. In 18 of the 29 states in the country, there has been a perceptible shift in focus on male sterilization. The state of Gujarat experienced a 20-fold increase in the annual number of vasectomies performed (**Fig. 6**). (S.K. Sikdar, MBBS, personal communication, December 12, 2008.). The increased uptake of vasectomy coincided with a revised compensation plan for vasectomy acceptors ands providers.

Except for Bhutan and Iran, vasectomy prevalence in Asia has declined steadily over the past 15 years (**Fig. 7**). In Bhutan and Iran, the government is making a special effort to promote and increase access to vasectomy. In Bhutan, the King has issued messages promoting male involvement in family planning. Vasectomy

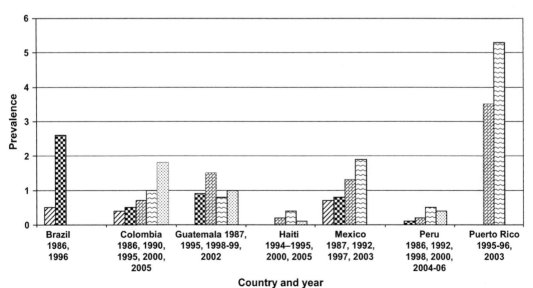

Fig. 3. Trends in vasectomy prevalence in Latin America and the Caribbean among currently married women aged 15 to 49, selected countries, 1986 to 2006. (*Data from* Refs.[1,6,25].)

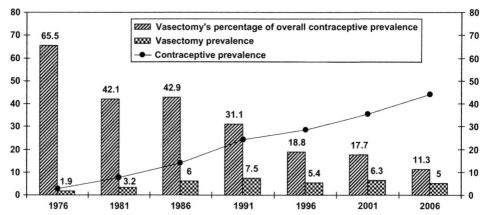

Fig. 4. Decline in vasectomy's contribution to the modern method mix in Nepal (1976–2006). (*Data from* Measure DHS. MEASURE DHS STATCompiler. Available at: http://www.statcompiler.com/start.cfm?action=new_table& userid=262970&usertabid=285250&CFID=419779&CFTOKEN=93662272, Accessed January 9, 2009; and Pradhan A, Aryal RH, Regmi G, et al. Nepal: family health survey 1996. Kathmandu and Calverton [MD]: Ministry of Health [Nepal], New Era and Macro International; 1997.)

services are free and mobile teams ensure rural areas have access to vasectomy services. In Iran, the public health system vigorously encourages private sector physicians to offer vasectomy. They are provided free training and instruments and are contracted to provide services in the public sector.[24]

Vasectomy in Africa

Although vasectomy services have been introduced within several sub-Saharan African countries, including Ghana, Kenya, Malawi, Rwanda, and Tanzania, in much of Africa, vasectomy prevalence rarely exceeds 0.1% and has remained relatively constant over the past decade.[25] Researchers have suggested that vasectomy is unacceptable to most African men and probably will long remain so.[26,27] Similar predictions in the late 1980s, however, that female sterilization would never be an acceptable method[28] proved unfounded.[29]

CHARACTERISTICS OF VASECTOMY ACCEPTORS

The profile of vasectomy acceptors in the developed and developing world varies significantly by

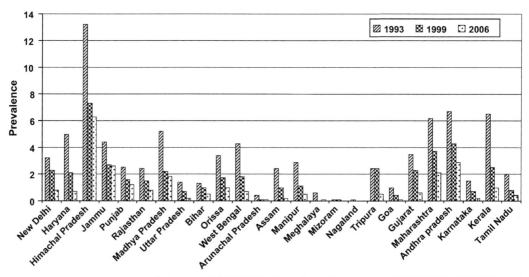

Fig. 5. Vasectomy prevalence in India by state (1993–2006). (*Data from* Measure DHS. MEASURE DHS STATCompiler. Available at: http://www.statcompiler.com/start.cfm?action=new_table&userid=262970&usertabid=285250& CFID=419779&CFTOKEN=93662272, Accessed January 9, 2009.)

State	2006-07	2007-08	Increase
Gujarat	1,032	20,646	20-fold
West Bengal	1,828	18,352	10-fold
Bihar	1,134	6,238	5 ½-fold
Jammu & Kashmir	404	1,879	4 ½-fold
Madhya Pradesh	10,972	30,816	3-fold
Orissa	790	2,605	3-fold
Jharkhand	6,461	17,281	2 ¾-fold
Delhi	1,320	3,467	2 ½-fold
Punjab	5,615	11,048	2-fold
Himachal Pradesh	3,144	5,289	1 ¾-fold

Fig. 6. States whose performance in NSV substantially improved in 2007 to 2008 over 2006 to 2007. (*Data from* S.K. Sikdar, MBBS, Joint Director, Monitoring and Evaluation Division, Ministry of Health and Family Welfare, Government of India. Increase in vasectomy acceptance in India, personal communication, December 12, 2008.)

region. Standardized population-based surveys, such as Demographic and Health Surveys provide insight into the characteristics of sterilization users. The most common data available include average age of the vasectomy users or partners, the number of children, education level, where the couples live, and where vasectomy procedures were performed.

United States and Canada

There is limited information on the characteristics of men receiving vasectomy in the United States. A nationwide study conducted in 1998 to1999 found that despite the diversity of the US population, men who have a vasectomy tended to be a homogeneous group, primarily non-Hispanic white men who are well educated, married, relatively affluent, and privately insured.[30] Minority, low-income, and less educated men made up

a disproportionately small share of vasectomy clients. Data gathered from men in the 2002 cycle of the NSFG reveal similar findings. For example, although 8% of men aged 15 to 44 reported having a vasectomy, only 2.3% of Hispanic/Latino men and 1.9 % of black/African American men reported the same.[19] In addition, the percentage of married men reporting they had a vasectomy was more than twice that of all men in the same age group that reported they had a vasectomy (13.3% versus 6.2%).[19] Men in the 300% of the poverty level or higher group were 2.5 times more likely to report having had a vasectomy compared to men in the 0 to 99% level.[19]

Demographic and socioeconomic profiles among sterilized women in the United States essentially are the reverse of those among vasectomized men. For example, data from the 2002 NSFG (as reported by women and men about their own and their partner's sterilization status) show

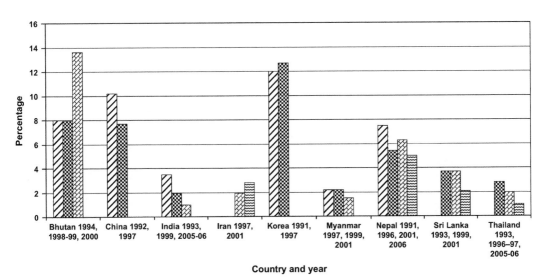

Fig. 7. Trends in vasectomy prevalence in Asia among currently married women aged 15 to 49, selected countries, 1991 to 2006. (*Data from* Refs.[1,11,12,25].)

that women who have had a tubal sterilization tend to be less educated and poorer than men who have had a vasectomy.[18,19] Sometimes, the differences are striking. For example, among women currently using contraception, 55.2% of women with a tubal sterilization had no high school diploma or General Educational Development high school equivalency, whereas at this same educational level only 2.8% of women reported that their partner had a vasectomy.[18] Likewise, among the poorest women (0–99% of the poverty level), 42.1% reported having had a tubal sterilization, whereas only 4.9% reported they rely on vasectomy for sterilization.[18] In addition, more black/African American and Hispanic/Latina women have had a tubal ligation compared to white women—opposite the pattern seen among vasectomized men (**Fig. 8**).[18,19]

Several studies have found that men in United States chose sterilization over temporary contraceptive methods because they believed it was the most secure family planning method, they or their partner disliked other methods, it was permanent, or they had a recent unplanned pregnancy or pregnancy scare.[30–32] In the 2002 NSFG, the vast majority of women who reported that their husband or cohabiting partner had a vasectomy cited not wanting any more children as the main reason for choosing vasectomy.[18] Men, women, and couples report that they specifically chose vasectomy over tubal ligation because it is safer and simpler, with shorter recovery time, and, to a lesser extent, men wanted to take responsibility for pregnancy prevention.[30–33]

Urologists are the main providers of vasectomy in the United States, performing 79% of all vasectomies in 2002, with 13% performed by family physicians and 8% by general surgeons.[34] Use of the no-scalpel vasectomy (NSV) approach to the vas increased in the United States between 1995 and 2002; 29% of vasectomies done in 1995 were NSV[34] compared with 48% of those performed in 2002.[34] In addition, the number of physicians who reported they currently performed NSV increased between 1995 and 2002, from 23% to 38%.[16,19] Wide variation is seen in occlusion methods and follow-up protocols used by physicians in the United States providing vasectomy services.[16,34,35]

Family medicine physicians are a significant provider of vasectomy in Canada—in 2005 to 2006, they performed 43% of all vasectomies, with the remaining 57% performed by surgical specialists (although no further breakdown of the latter is provided, it is likely that most of these were done by urologists or general surgeons).[20]

Latin America

Studies in Brazil, Colombia, and Mexico indicate that a "typical" vasectomy acceptor is in his mid-30s, has an educational level higher than the national average, has had three or fewer children, lives in an urban area, and has used other contraceptive methods before choosing vasectomy.[36,37] According to this profile, men are having vasectomies at an earlier age and after they have had fewer children, on average, than acceptors from the 1980s, when vasectomy services first became available.[36,38]

Among vasectomy acceptors interviewed in population-based studies, the overwhelming majority lived in urban areas. For example, in Brazil, Guatemala, and Mexico, 90% of vasectomy acceptors lived in urban areas; in Colombia, 80% of couples who were protected by vasectomy lived in urban areas, as did 67% of such couples in Peru. Other than in El Salvador and Mexico, most vasectomy procedures in the 1980s were performed by private providers and nongovernmental organizations, such as Pro-Pater (Brazil), Profamilia (Colombia), and APROFAM (Guatemala). Over the past decade, however, the role of the public sector in providing vasectomy has increased in several countries (**Fig. 9**), although the public sector accounts for less than

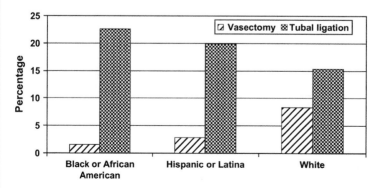

Fig. 8. Use of sterilization among women aged 15 to 44 in the United States, 2002. (*Data from* Chandra A, Martinez GM, Mosher WD, et al. Fertility, family planning, and reproductive health of U.S. women: data from the 2002 National survey of family growth. National center for health statistics. Vital Health Stat 2005;23[25].)

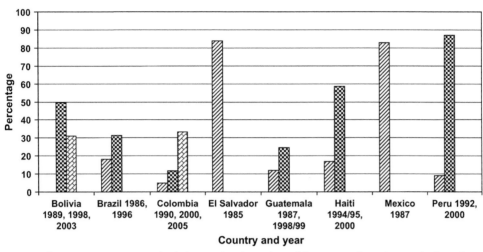

Fig. 9. Percent of vasectomy acceptors obtaining services from the public sector, selected countries in Latin America, 1986 to 2005. (*Data from* Measure DHS. MEASURE DHS STATCompiler. Available at: http://www.statcompiler.com/start.cfm?action=new_table&userid=262970&usertabid=285250&CFID=419779&CFTOKEN=93662272. Accessed January 9, 2009.)

50% of vasectomies. Exceptions are Haiti and Peru and countries that have longstanding public sector programs, such as El Salvador and Mexico.

Asia

For a "typical" Asian couple using vasectomy, the wife is in her mid- to late 30s and has little or no education. The couple has three or more children and lives in a rural area. In most Asian countries, men have had their vasectomy performed at a public sector facility. (Unless otherwise noted, information in this section has been extracted from country-level demographic health surveys.)[25]

In Indonesia and Nepal, three out of four wives of vasectomy acceptors interviewed were 35 years old or older, whereas in India four out of five such women and in Sri Lanka three out of five were 35years old or older. In Indonesia and Nepal, approximately half of vasectomy acceptors had four or more children, whereas in India, the Philippines, and Thailand, approximately 33% of vasectomy acceptors had three children. Sri Lanka (30%) and Thailand (35%) had a sizable number of vasectomy acceptors who had only two children.

In India (62%) and Nepal (81%), the majority of women whose husbands had vasectomies had no education, whereas the majority of such women in Indonesia (59%) and Thailand (73%) had a primary education. The majority of women whose husbands had vasectomies had a secondary or higher education in Sri Lanka (52%). In Indonesia, Nepal, Sri Lanka, and Thailand, four out of five vasectomy acceptors lived in rural areas, whereas in India and the Philippines three out of four and two out of three acceptors, respectively, lived in rural areas.

In Indonesia and the Philippines, the proportion of couples reporting their vasectomy procedure had been performed in a public sector facility declined through the late 1980s but has since risen slightly. For example, in Indonesia, between 1987 and 1997, the proportion of vasectomies performed in the public sector declined from 96% to 87%, whereas from 1997 to 2002 there was a slight increase from 87% to 92%. Likewise, in the Philippines, after the proportion of vasectomies performed in the public sector declined from 57% in 1993 to 47% in 1998, the proportion increased over 30 percentage points to 79.2% between 1998 and 2003.

Sub-Saharan Africa

Because the prevalence of vasectomy is negligible in Africa, population-based studies do not shed much light on the characteristics of vasectomy acceptors there. Studies of vasectomy acceptors in Kenya, Rwanda, and Tanzania in the early and mid-1990s indicated that the typical acceptor was in his late 30s or early 40s, had some secondary education, had used family planning methods in the past, and had had five or more children. In addition, he most likely had the procedure performed at a private or nongovernmental organization facility.[39–41] Recent data from Ghana revealed the average vasectomy acceptor was 44 years old and had four children.[42] A marketing campaign and vasectomy service introduction program targeted at men in Nairobi suggested that the profile of the urban vasectomy acceptor in Kenya may be changing, however. Acceptors were younger (in their mid- to late 30s) and had fewer children (3.2). They also were better educated: 90% had attained at least a high school education, and 85% were professionals (eg, high school teachers or civil servants).[43]

SUMMARY

Vasectomy often is ignored, despite its being one of the safest, simplest, most highly effective, and least-expensive contraceptive methods. Vasectomy remains the family planning method that is least known, understood, or used, a fact confirmed in Demographic and Health Survey studies conducted in 21 countries over the past 5 years. Men in every part of the world and every cultural, religious, or socioeconomic setting have demonstrated interest in or acceptance of vasectomy despite commonly held assumptions about negative male attitudes or societal prohibitions. Because men lack full access to information and services, however, they cannot make informed decisions or take an active part in family planning.

REFERENCES

1. United Nations. World contraceptive use 2007 (wall chart). New York: United Nations, Department of Economic and Social Affairs, Population Division; 2008.
2. Population Reference Bureau. Family planning worldwide 2008 data sheet. Washington, D.C: Population Reference Bureau; 2008.
3. Bensyl D, Iuliano D, Carter M, et al. Contraceptive use—United States and territories, behavioral risk factor surveillance system, 2002. MMWR Surveill Summ 2005;54(6):1–72.
4. Bangladesh Ministry of Health and family Welfare, National Institute for Populations Research and Training (NIPORT), Mitra and Associates Opinion Research Corp. MEASURE DHS Macro International Inc. Bangladesh DHS—preliminary report 2007. Calverton (MD): Macro International; December 2007.
5. Secretaria de Salud. Encuestra Nacional de Salud Reproducitva 2003: tabulados Basica. Mexico: Secretaria de Salud, Centro Regional de Investigaciones Multidisciplanarias UNAM; 2006.
6. Institute National de la Statistique Ministere de la Planifacation Economique et des Finances, Ministere de la Sante, Macro International. Rwanda Enquete Intemediare demographique et sante 20007-2008: rapport preliminaire. Calverron (MD), USA: Macro International; 2008.
7. Office for National Statistics [United Kingdom]. Omnibus survey report no. 37: Contraception and sexual health 2007/08. Norwich (UK): Office of Public Sector Information; 2008.
8. Liskin L, Pile JM, Quillan WF. Vasectomy—safe and simple. Population reports, series D, no. 4. Baltimore (MD): Johns Hopkins University, Population Information Program; 1983.
9. Liskin L, Benoit E, Blackburn R. Vasectomy: new opportunities. Population reports, series D, no. 5. Baltimore (MD): Johns Hopkins University, Population Information Program; 1992.
10. EngenderHealth. Contraceptive sterilization. New York: global issues and trends; 2002.
11. UN. World contraceptive use, 2001 (wall chart). New York: United Nations, Department of Economic and Social Affairs, Population Division; 2002.
12. UN. World contraceptive use, 2005 (wall chart). New York: United Nations, Department of Economic and Social Affairs, Population Division; 2006.
13. Piccinino LJ, Mosher WD. Trends in contraceptive use in the United States: 1982–1995. Fam Plann Perspect 1998;30(1):4–10 46.
14. Chandra AA. No. 20In: Surgical sterilization in the United States: prevalence and characteristics, 1965–95, Vital and Health Statistics, vol. 23. Hyattsville (MD): National Center for Health Statistics; 1998.
15. Magnani RJ, Haws JM, Morgan GT, et al. Vasectomy in the United States, 1991 and 1995. Am J Public Health 1999;89(1):92–4.
16. Barone MA, Hutchinson PL, Johnson CH, et al. Vasectomy in the United States, 2002. J Urol 2006; 176(1):232–6.
17. Mosher WD, Martinez GM, Chandra A, et al. Use of contraception and use of family planning services in the United States: 1982–2002. Advance data from vital and health statistics. No. 350. Hyattsville (MD): National Center for Health Statistics; 2004.
18. Chandra A, Martinez GM, Mosher WD, et al. Fertility, family planning, and reproductive health of U.S. women: data from the 2002 National survey of family growth. National center for health statistics. Vital Health Stat 2005;23(25).
19. Martinez GM, Chandra A, Abma JC, et al. Fertility, contraception, and fatherhood: Data on men and women from Cycle 6 (2002) of the national survey of family growth. National center for health statistics. Vital Health Stat 2006;23(26).
20. Canadian Institute for Health Information (CIHI). Physicians in Canada: fee-for-service utilization, 2005–2006. Ottawa: CIHI; 2008.
21. Statistics Canada. Profile of age and sex for Canada, provinces, territories, census divisions and census subdivisions, 2006 census. Statistics Canada; 2007.
22. Sneyd MJ, Cox B, Paul C, et al. High prevalence of vasectomy in New Zealand. Contraception 2001; 64(3):155–9.
23. Santow G. Trends in contraception and sterilization in Australia. Aust N Z J Obstet Gynaecol 1991;31(3): 201–8.

24. Kols A, Lande R. Vasectomy: reaching out to new users. Population reports, series D, no.6. Baltimore (MD): INFO Project, Johns Hopkins Schol of Public Health; June 2008.

25. Measure DHS. MEASURE DHS STATcompiler. Available at: http://www.statcompiler.com/start.cfm?action=new_table&userid=262970&usertabid=285250&CFID=419779&CFTOKEN=93662272. Accessed January 9, 2009.

26. Ross JA, Hong S, Huber D. Voluntary sterilization: an international fact book. New York: Association for Voluntary Sterilization; 1985.

27. Caldwell JC, Caldwell P. Africa: the new family planning frontier. Stud Fam Plann 2002;33(1):76–86.

28. Caldwell JC, Caldwell P. The cultural context of high fertility in sub-Saharan Africa. Popul Dev Rev 1987; 13(3):409–37.

29. Dwyer JC, Haws JM. Is permanent contraception acceptable in sub-Saharan Africa? Stud Fam Plann 1990;21(6):322–6.

30. Barone MA, Johnson CH, Luick MA, et al. Characteristics of men receiving vasectomies in the United States, 1998-1999. Perspect Sex Reprod Health 2004;36:27–33.

31. Landry E, Ward V. Perspectives from couples on the vasectomy decision: a six-country study. In: Ravindran TKS, Berer M, Cottingham J, editors. Beyond acceptability: users' perspectives on contraception. London: Reproductive Health Matters; 1997. p. 58–67.

32. Philliber SG, Philliber WW. Social and psychological perspectives on voluntary sterilization: a review. Stud Fam Plann 1985;16(1):1–29.

33. Shain RN, Pasta DJ. Tubal sterilization or vasectomy: how do married couples make the choice? Fertil Steril 1991;56(2):278–84.

34. Haws JM, Morgan GT, Pollack AE, et al. Clinical aspects of vasectomies performed in the United States in 1995. Urology 1998;52:685–91.

35. Deneux-Tharaux C, Kahn E, Nazerali H, et al. Pregnancy rates after vasectomy: a survey of US urologists. Contraception 2004;69:401–6.

36. Alarcon F, Juarez C, Ward V, et al. Vasectomy decision-making in Mexico (GLO-11-EV-1): a global vasectomy decision-making study: a six-part series. New York: AVSC International; 1995.

37. Vernon R. Operations research on promoting vasectomy in three Latin American countries. Int Fam Plann Persp 1996;22(1):26–31.

38. Santiso R, Bertrand JT, Pineda MA. Voluntary sterilization in Guatemala: a comparison of men and women. Stud Fam Plann 1983;14(3):73–82.

39. Binyange M, Cyridion U, Ward V, et al. Vasectomy decision-making in Rwanda. New York: Association for Voluntary Surgical Contraception; 1993.

40. Lynam P, Dwyer J, Wilkinson D, et al. Vasectomy in Kenya: the first steps. AVSC working paper number 4. New York: AVSC; 1993.

41. Muhondwa E, Rutenberg N. Effects of the vasectomy promotion project on knowledge, attitudes and behavior among men in Dar es Salaam, Tanzania, Nairobi, Kenya. Operation Research Technical Assistance Africa Project II; 1997 [Report].

42. The ACQUIRE Project. Get a permanent smile'-increasing awareness of, access to, and utilization of vasectomy services in Ghana. New York: The ACQUIRE Project/EngenderHealth; 2005.

43. Ruminjo K, Adriance D, Pile JM. Social marketing of vasectomy—a pilot project to increase the availability and accessibility of no-scalpel vasectomy services in Nairobi, Kenya. New York: EngenderHealth; 2002.

Techniques of Vasectomy

Kevin S. Art, MD, Ajay K. Nangia, MBBS*

KEYWORDS

- Vasectomy • Male contraception
- Vasal occlusion • Technique • Vas deferens

Vasectomy is the most commonly performed urologic surgical procedure performed in the United States. An estimated 500,000 men undergo the procedure each year in the United States,[1] equivalent to 11% of all married couples relying on vasectomy for contraception.[2] The widespread use of vasectomy is mirrored by wide variations in surgical techniques, follow-up protocols, and procedural costs. This article discusses key aspects of surgical anatomy, preoperative considerations, commonly used surgical techniques, and postoperative care.

PATIENT COUNSELING

As with any surgical procedure, vasectomy should be performed only after thorough patient counseling is performed. It is ideal if both partners participate in the counseling session. As suggested by Schwingl and Guess, alternative methods of contraception, the intended irreversible nature of vasectomy, and risk for failure should be discussed with each patient.[2] Other risks, including the incidence of chronic pain, should be discussed. A surgeon may be confronted with unique ethical issues, such as unilateral decision making (ie, only the male partner making the decision without his partner involved), young age of the patient, and so forth. These possible scenarios underscore the need for a detailed conversation with each individual patient. Fully informed consent should be obtained only after discussing the risks for the procedure and alternative forms of therapy.

Despite the intended irreversibility of the procedure, up to 6% of men who undergo vasectomy request vasectomy reversal.[3] The most common reasons cited by patients seeking vasectomy reversal include divorce and remarriage.[4,5] Several investigators have shown that men younger than age 30 at the time of vasectomy are 12 times more likely to seek vasectomy reversal in the future than those who underwent vasectomy after age 30.[3,6] Should a patient inquire about the possibility of reversal to regain fertility in the future, a surgeon should carefully discuss the risks and variable success rates of the procedure and its possible cost. Prevasectomy sperm cryopreservation remains an option, although its cost-effectiveness is debatable and may suggest a patient's indecision about permanent contraception. This should be discussed with patients if they request.

SURGICAL ANATOMY

A proper understanding of surgical anatomy lies at the foundation of any successful surgical procedure. The different layers of the scrotum and the course of the vas as it ascends from the scrotum are key points for physicians performing a vasectomy.

Scrotal Tissue Layers

The scrotum contains the testes, epididymis, and portions of the vas deferens. It is divided into halves by the scrotal septum, which is denoted by the median raphe on the scrotal skin. The skin of the scrotum itself is hirsute and contains many sebaceous glands. The scrotal skin is firmly attached to the underlying superficial fascial layer, known as dartos fascia. Deep to the dartos fascia is the external spermatic fascia, which is

Department of Urology, University of Kansas Medical Center, Mailstop 3016, 3901 Rainbow Boulevard, Kansas City, KS 66160, USA

* Corresponding author.

E-mail address: anangia@kumc.edu (A.K. Nangia).

Urol Clin N Am 36 (2009) 307–316

doi:10.1016/j.ucl.2009.05.005

a continuation of the external muscle fascia of the abdominal wall. The external spermatic fascia is continuous over the penis as Buck's fascia. The internal oblique muscle of the abdominal wall gives rise to the cremasteric muscle and fascia. Deep to the cremaster lays the internal spermatic fascia, which is derived from the transversalis fascia. The vas deferens is reached once the internal spermatic fascia is opened. The relationship of scrotal tissue layers in relation to the vas is demonstrated in **Fig. 1**.

Anatomic variations of scrotal anatomy also must be considered when performing vasectomy. In the majority of patients, vasectomy is performed outside of the tunica vaginalis. Autopsy studies show, however, that approximately 12% of men have high insertions of the tunica vaginalis (bell-clapper deformity).[7] In these patients, the tunica vaginalis completely encircles the testis, epididymis, and distal spermatic cord (including the vas). Vasectomy performed in patients who have this variant is, therefore, inside the tunica vaginalis and potentially leads to the development of a hydrocele in some cases.

Vasal Anatomy

Spanning a length of approximately 45 cm, the vas deferens (ductus deferens) connects the testicle to the seminal vesicles, which coalesces with the vasal ampulla to become the ejaculatory ducts. The vas begins at the epididymal tail (globus minor) as the convoluted vas. It is a thick-walled tube consisting of mucosal and submucosal layers surrounded by an outer longitudinal and inner circular smooth muscle.[8] As the vas begins its ascent within the scrotum, it travels medially to the epididymis and then posteriorly as it enters the spermatic cord. It is in this region of the scrotum where the vas can be palpated as a firm cord close to the pampiniform plexus. Once above

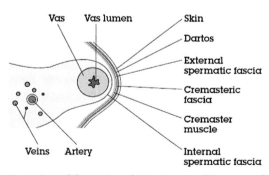

Fig. 1. Scrotal layers in relation to vas. (*Courtesy of* EngenderHealth, New York, NY; with permission. Copyright © 2008. This material is taken from EngenderHealth's "No-scalpel vasectomy: an illustrated guide for surgeons" 3rd ed.)

the testicle, the vas becomes straight as it ascends within the spermatic cord posterior to the cord vessels. Occasionally it can be palpated anteriorly. After the vas passes through the inguinal canal, it emerges in the pelvis lateral to the inferior epigastric vessels.[8] It then passes medially to the other pelvic side wall structures and enters the prostatic base posteriorly. At the terminal end of the vas is the ampulla—a tortuous and dilated segment that is able to store spermatozoa.

Blood Supply

The vas receives it blood from the deferential artery—a branch of the inferior vesical artery. Anastomoses between the testicular artery and deferential artery provide collateral circulation to the structures. The cremasteric artery (branch of the inferior epigastric artery) also often participates in the collateral circulation.

OPERATIVE CONSIDERATIONS
Antimicrobial Prophylaxis

The scrotum generally is classified as clean-contaminated because of its close proximity to the perineum.[9] Despite the proximity to the perineum, the incidence of surgical site infection (SSI) after conventional incisional vasectomy or the no-scapel vasectomy (NSV) is low, ranging from 1.5% to 9%.[10–12] For this reason, prophylactic antimicrobials typically are not used when performing vasectomy, especially when performed in the clinic setting.[13] Additionally, the use of prophylactic antibiotics for the prevention of bacterial endocarditis no longer is recommended during urologic procedures.[14] A recent advisory council, however, has recommended the use of prophylactic antibiotic use in select patients who have total joint replacements. These patients include those who have had joint replacements within the past 2 years, are immunocompromised or -suppressed, or who have additional comorbidities, such as HIV, diabetes, malignancy, or prior joint replacement infections.[15]

There are no randomized controlled studies on the use of prophylactic antibiotics with vasectomies but many reports on infectious complications from vasectomy. Many high-volume practices do not use antibiotics but if surgeons prefer the use of prophylactic antibiotics, they should be aimed at preventing infection from common pathogens of the genitourinary tract (*Escherichia coli*, *Proteus* sp, *Klepsiella* sp, and enterococcus) and skin (*Staphylococcus aureus*, coagulase-negative *Staphylococcus* sp, and group A streptococci sp).[13] Common choices for SSI prophylaxis during scrotal surgery include a first-generation cephalo-sporin (eg, cephalexin), fluoroquinolone (eg, levo-floxacin), or aminoglycoside (eg, gentamicin). These medications have appropriately long half-lives, are inexpensive when used as a single dose, and rarely are associated with allergic reactions.[13] Fluoroquinolones or aminoglycosides may be used when patients have a β-lactam allergy. Timing of administration is key; antibiotic should begin within 1 to 2 hours of incision.

Although preoperative antibiotics typically are not used in vasectomy, proper preoperative skin preparation is essential in reducing the risk for SSI. Hair removal often is necessary owing to the hirsute nature of the scrotal skin. Once appropriate hair removal is completed, antiseptic solutions are applied to the surgical site. Typically, chlorhexi-dine-based antiseptics or povidone-iodine are used.[16]

Anesthesia

The majority of vasectomies performed in the United States are done under local anesthesia in a clinic setting. Local anesthesia is safer than general anesthesia and more cost effective. The initial puncture of the scrotal skin with the needle to inject anesthetic agents, however, often is the greatest source of anxiety for patients. The use of eutectic mixture of local anesthetics (EMLA) cream for topical anesthetic to minimize discomfort of the needle puncture has been advocated.[17,18] The efficacy of this practice, however, recently has come under scrutiny.[19] An oral sedative, such as diazepam, often is given 1 hour before the procedure to relax patients. This in turn aids in relaxing scrotal musculature and facilitates the procedure.[20]

To perform needle injection, the vas is brought to the scrotal surface using a three-finger technique, as described by Li and colleagues[21,22] It is essential to isolate the vas away from the vessels of the spermatic cord and the base of the penis. Local vasal nerve block is achieved with 1% to 2% lidocaine without epinephrine in a 1.5-in, 25-gauge needle. An alternative solution can be used with a 1:1 ratio of 1% lidocaine and 0.5% bupivicaine.[20] The authors use a mixture of chloroprocaine and bupivicaine in a 1:1 ratio. Chloroprocaine has a rapid onset of action (quicker than lidocaine) and has no burning effect on injection but has a short half-life of 30 minutes. A subcutaneous wheal is raised at the scrotal skin surface. The needle is advanced within the perivasal sheath and approximately 2 to 3 mL of anesthetic is injected around the vas (**Fig. 2**). It is essential to avoid excessive needle movement or

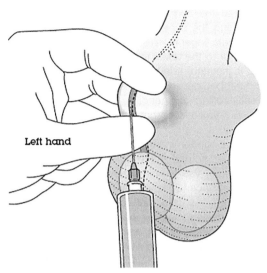

Fig. 2. Three-finger grasp used to inject anesthetic. (*Courtesy of* EngenderHealth, New York, NY; with permission. Copyright © 2008. This material is taken from EngenderHealth's "No-scalpel vasectomy: an illustrated guide for surgeons" 3rd ed.)

multiple punctures as this increases the risk for hematoma formation and can impair vas exposure due to edema.[20,23]

The recent innovation of no-needle vasectomy, as described by Weiss and Li and Monoski and colleagues, uses a jet injection technique to establish local anesthesia. A jet injection instrument generates a high-pressure spray, which is forced through the skin, vas, and perivasal tissues.[21,24] Reported advantages of this method of local anesthesia include decreased tissue trauma, faster onset of action, and decreased volume of solution required for local anesthesia.[24]

APPROACHING THE VAS

Access to the vas and its delivery from the scrotum is the first component of vasectomy, regardless of the method of vasal occlusion used. This often is the most difficult aspect of the procedure for less-experienced surgeons. Before any incision or percutaneous entry of the scrotum is performed, the vas first must be isolated from other spermatic cord structures. Ideally, the vas should be isolated away from the base of the penis and in the midscrotal vas region to prevent possible testicular or inguinal pain during or after the procedure. This is made easier if the scrotum is relaxed (relaxed patient in a warm environment). The three-finger technique, also known as the tripod-grasp, is a common method for isolating the vas. The nondominant thumb is placed on the median raphe at the midpoint between the base of the penis and the superior margin of the testis. The left middle finger then is used to probe the scrotum posterior to the testis to locate the vas. Once the vas is isolated, it is brought anterior to the testis and trapped between the thumb and middle finger. Gently rolling or kneading the vas between the fingers helps ensure that other vessels of the spermatic cord are not trapped along with the vas. Next, the nondominant index finger is swept gently over the scrotal skin overlying the trapped segment of vas to minimize the tissue from the scrotal surface to the vas itself. Once the segment is isolated, the dominant hand is used to administer a local vasal nerve block or apply the jet injection technique. After sufficient anesthesia is induced, the operating surgeon may proceed to penetrate the overlying scrotal skin through a conventional incision or via the no-scalpel technique.

VASECTOMY TECHNIQUES
Conventional Incision Technique

In the conventional technique, bilateral 1-cm transverse incisions are made in the scrotal skin using a no. 15 blade scalpel. The incisions are carried down through the vasal sheath until the vas is reached. The vas then is delivered from the surrounding sheath while the deferential artery and nerves are isolated and swept away. The vas is transected and a length of vas is excised. This segment may range from 0 to 4 cm in length.[25] The ends of the vas are occluded by one of several possible methods. These options for occlusion of the vas are discussed later. Once the vasectomy is completed, the scrotal skin typically is closed with absorbable sutures. Topical antibiotic ointment often is applied to the incision site and fluffed gauze dressings are applied.

No-scalpel Vasectomy

The NSV technique was first described by Li and colleagues in 1974.[23] NSV eliminates the need for scrotal skin incision, which may contribute to its lower incidence of scrotal hematomas and infections.[11]

In the NSV technique, a vasal nerve block is performed (described previously). Once the vas is isolated using the nondominant hand, a ring-tipped fixation clamp is opened and pressed downward into the scrotal skin. By opening the tips of the fixation clamp as it is pressed into the scrotal skin, the skin is overlying the vas stretched tightly around the vas as it is secured in the ring (**Fig. 3**). A sharp-tip curved mosquito hemostat then punctures the scrotal skin through the same puncture hole created by the needle used for local anesthesia (**Fig. 4**). The ringed fixation clamp is advanced into the opening and the vas is grasped and delivered.[20]

The bare vas is isolated by stripping the surrounding layers using a sharp-tip hemostat. The blade of the hemostat that punctured the vas wall is used to divide the vas from the lumen outward while the ringed clamp is rotated 180°, a process known as the "supination maneuver," thereby delivering the vas through the puncture hole. The ring clamp then is used to secure the vas outside of the scrotal skin. The sharp-tip hemostat is used to clean the vas vessels and isolate an appropriate segment of bare vas (**Fig. 5**). If desired, a scalpel may be used to incise the vas sheath rather than the sharp hemostat. Once the bare vas segment is isolated, it is divided and occluded. This technique is repeated on the contralateral side.

Modified No-scalpel Vasectomy

In a typical NSV, the sharp hemostat is designed to spear the vas and lift it through the wound by

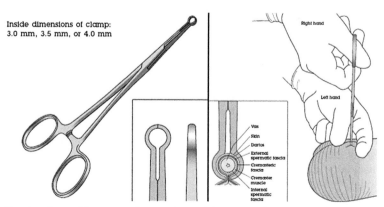

Inside dimensions of clamp: 3.0 mm, 3.5 mm, or 4.0 mm

Fig. 3. Ringed-tip fixation clamp. (*Courtesy of* EngenderHealth, New York, NY; with permission. Copyright © 2008. This material is taken from EngenderHealth's "No-scalpel vasectomy: an illustrated guide for surgeons" 3rd ed.)

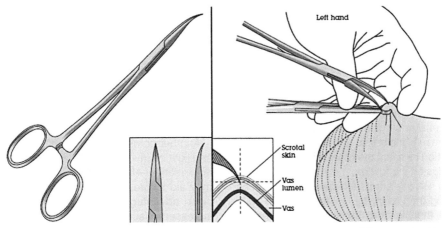

Fig. 4. Sharp-t. (*Courtesy of* EngenderHealth, New York, NY; with permission. Copyright © 2008. This material is taken from EngenderHealth's "No-scalpel vasectomy: an illustrated guide for surgeons" 3rd ed.)

rotating the wrist 180° (supination maneuver). Jones developed a simple modification to the NSV to avoid the supination maneuver, which is, along with fixation of the vas, often cited as one of the most difficult aspect of the NSV to master.[26] Rather than fixing the vas to the skin with the ringed fixation clamp, the ulnar prong of the sharp hemostat is placed through the skin all the way to the vas while it is secured in the three-finger grasp of the nondominant hand. The clamp is closed and placed through the incision and spread to expose the vas. The ringed clamp is placed through the incision and secured around the vas, facilitating its delivery through the skin. Surgeons may perform vasal excision and occlusion by their method of choice.

METHODS OF VASAL OCCLUSION

Regardless of the method used to access the vas, the second step of any vasectomy is disruption of the vas. The choice of occlusion varies between surgeons and is independent of which method is used to approach the vas. Materials and techniques commonly used include suture ligature, surgical clips, thermal or electrocautery, intra vas devices, vas excision, open-end vasectomy, and fascial interposition.[27] These techniques often are used in varying combinations for vas occlusion. The method used for occlusion the vas may determine the incidence of recanalization and subsequent vasectomy failure.

Excision and Ligation

Excision of a segment of vas commonly is performed to minimize the risk for recanalization, although no standard minimum of length has been established. Labrecque and colleagues[28] studied a cohort of 870 men to determine if an association between length of the vas excised and risk

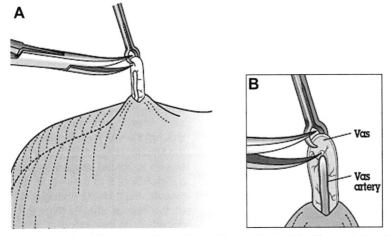

Fig. 5. Delivery and stripping of vas. (*Courtesy of* EngenderHealth, New York, NY; with permission. Copyright © 2008. This material is taken from EngenderHealth's "No-scalpel vasectomy: an illustrated guide for surgeons" 3rd ed.)

for recanalization existed. Segments of vas excised in this cohort ranged from 5 to 20 mm and all vas occlusions were performed using hemoclips. They determined that excising longer segments with a range of 5 to 20 mm does not reduce the risk for recanalization. The investigators of this article recommend excising a 1-cm segment.

Ligation of the vas ends may be performed with suture material or surgical clips. Suturing the ends of the vas results in fibrosis and scarring. Although suture ligation remains the most common method of vas occlusion worldwide,[20] trends in the United States vary. Barone studied the preferred methods of occluding the vas in the United States in 2002 and found that ligation only was performed by 16.9% of physicians whereas clips were used in only 8.8% of vasectomies.[1] Suture materials commonly used for ligation include silk, Vicryl, and chromic catgut. Special consideration of suture diameter also is warranted. Typically, 3-0 or 4-0 suture is used. Larger suture may interfere with the ability to perform fascial interposition (if desired) whereas many surgeons avoid using finer suture material for fear it may cut through the vas entirely leading to recanalization.[29] An adequate stump (approximately 3 mm) will help prevent the suture from sliding off the excised end (**Fig. 6**).

The use of surgical clips first was introduced by Gupta and coworkers in 1977.[30] For vasal occlusion, two hemoclips are placed approximately 1 cm apart before incision of the vas. Currently, less than 9% of surgeons in the United States use clips alone as a means of occlusion.[1] It is difficult to determine whether or not hemoclips offer decreased incidence of recanalization compared with nonabsorbable suture. Suture ligation of vasal

ends may lead to tissue necrosis and subsequent sloughing of the cut end distal to the ligature. If this occurs on both ends, recanalization may occur. Some investigators believe that the wider diameter of medium hemoclips (versus suture) distributes pressure more evenly to the vasal wall thereby decreasing the risk for necrosis and sloughing.[20] Although the advantage of hemoclips over suture is debatable.

Another commonly used variation after excision and ligation involves the folding back the vas ends after ligation. Although some surgeons believe this may aid in preventing recanalization, there is no clear advantage of this practice in terms of increased effectiveness of vasectomy.[31]

Fascial Interposition

After the vas is occluded, many surgeons choose to place a layer of the vas sheath between the two cut ends of the vas—a technique known as fascial interposition. In this technique, a suture is used to keep the testicular end of the vas contained within the vas sheath while the nontesticular (prostatic) end remains outside.[32] Accurate identification of the vas sheath is necessary for this occlusion method. Care must be taken to not cause bleeding of the vasal vessels that often are still attached to the sheath. The addition of fascial interposition adds time and technical difficulty to a vasectomy procedure, but it is associated with decreased recanalization rates.[32,33] In a large, randomized controlled trial, the use of fascial interposition resulted in faster azoospermia and oligospermia levels on semen analysis and reduced vasectomy failures by approximately half compared with ligation and excision alone.[32]

When fascial interposition is planned, the suture ties on the nontesticular end of the vas should be left long enough to remain outside of the incision when the nontesticular end returns to the scrotum. This facilitates retrieval of this end for interposition. After excision and ligation of the vas ends are performed, the testicular and nontesticular ends are allowed to return to the scrotum through the incision. The nontesticular end suture is grasped and the end is delivered through the scrotal incision. The fascial sheath should form a collar around the vas with the testicular end still within the sheath. Using a hemoclip or suture, the fascial sheath is ligated around the nontesticular vas at a distance of 2 to 3 mm from its end (**Fig. 7**). This closure results in the nontesticular vas end outside of the fascial sheath (**Fig. 8**).[34] Although introduced as an innovation for excision and ligation, fascial interposition also may be used after intraluminal cautery for vasal occlusion.

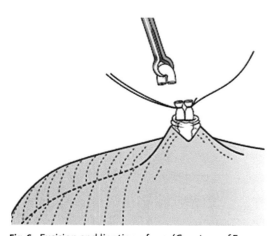

Fig. 6. Excision and ligation of vas. (*Courtesy of* EngenderHealth, New York, NY; with permission. Copyright © 2008. This material is taken from EngenderHealth's "No-scalpel vasectomy: an illustrated guide for surgeons" 3rd ed.)

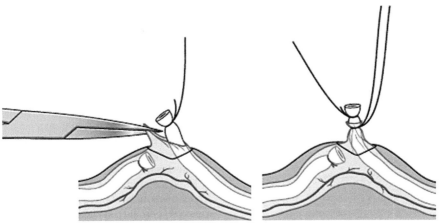

Fig. 7. Fascial interposition. (*Courtesy of* EngenderHealth, New York, NY; with permission. Copyright © 2008. This material is taken from EngenderHealth's "No-scalpel vasectomy: an illustrated guide for surgeons" 3rd ed.)

Cautery

Cautery is a highly effective method for occluding the vas during vasectomy. In the United States, cautery is the most commonly used method of vas occlusion, with more than 73% of surgeons using cautery alone or in combination with other methods,[1] reflecting a steady increase from 50% 10 years earlier.[35]

The principle of vas occlusion using cautery relies on adequate energy to destroy the vasal mucosa while minimizing damage to muscle layers. The cauterization technique is largely dependent of the equipment available to a surgeon. If a needlepoint electrode is used, the cold needle is used to pierce the vas wall and then directed into the lumen approximately 1 to 1.5 cm (**Fig. 9**). If a blunt-tip cautery is used, the vas needs to be hemitransected to allow the blunt electrode to enter the lumen. Once inside the lumen, current is applied and the electrode is slowly withdrawn. Surgeons should observe for blanching of the mucosa, which indicates tissue desiccation. The process is performed on the testicular and nontesticular ends of the vas. If cautery is applied for too long or at too high a current, the vasal muscle tissue may be damaged in addition to vasal mucosa. Such tissue damage increases the incidence of sperm leakage and recanalization.[34]

Electrocautery or thermal cautery may be used. Some surgeons prefer thermal cautery to electrocautery because it may result in lower incidence of granulomas and cause less nodular thickening of the vas. Also, histologic study has suggested that thermal cautery provides more reliable occlusion compared with electrocautery.[36] Several battery-powered devices are available for thermal cautery, which may be beneficial in settings where electricity is not readily unavailable.

Cautery Plus Fascial Interposition

Based on observed failure rates, vas occlusion methods that include the use of cautery are significantly more effective than those that do not.[33] Similarly, fascial interposition has been shown to improve the success of vasectomy when ligation and excision are used.[32] For these reasons, many investigators believe that cautery plus fascial interposition results in the lowest risk for recanalization. So far, evidence exists to support the combination of cautery and fascial interposition;[31] however, these findings are not conclusive.

Open-ended Vasectomy

Pressure-induced damage to the epididymis and pain is a potential consequence of vasectomy when the testicular end of the vas is occluded.[20]

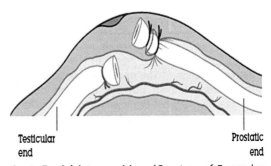

Testicular end   Prostatic end

Fig. 8. Fascial intersposition. (*Courtesy of* EngenderHealth, New York, NY; with permission. Copyright © 2008. This material is taken from EngenderHealth's "No-scalpel vasectomy: an illustrated guide for surgeons" 3rd ed.)

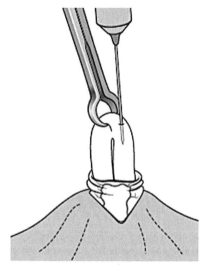

Fig. 9. Needle-tip cautery. (*Courtesy of* Engender-Health, New York, NY; with permission. Copyright © 2008. This material is taken from EngenderHealth's "No-scalpel vasectomy: an illustrated guide for surgeons" 3rd ed.)

This increased pressure is not transmitted to the seminiferous tubules; thus, little if any impact on spermatogenesis is observed.[37] If the testicular end of the vas is not occluded, leakage of sperm may occur resulting in the formation of a sperm granuloma at the vasectomy site. In theory, this process acts as a "pop-off" valve, which dissipates pressure and thereby may prevent damage to the epididymis—an important factor in successful vasectomy reversal.[38] Many surgeons prefer this technique to allow for sperm granuloma formation, which may in turn aid in successful reversal and prevent long-term orchalgia after vasectomy. Not surprisingly, open-ended techniques are associated with higher vasectomy failure rates compared with closed occlusion techniques.[20]

Intravasal Device (Experimental)

Vasectomy may result in vasitis nodosa, chronic testicular or epididymal pain, and alterations in testicular function.[20] The causes of these complications are unknown but are believed due to complete blockage of the vas. Researchers have sought to maintain duct patency to avoid these complications while preserving the contraceptive efficacy. This has lead to the development of the intravasal device (IVD).

Song and colleagues[39] published findings from a phase II randomized controlled trial comparing the efficacy and safety of the IVD to the NSV in 2006. The IVD is comprised of an outer shell composed of urethane and filled with nylon thread. Only 1 mm in outer diameter and 17 mm in length, the device can be inserted into the vas lumen through a mini-incision. There are two sulci near the head and tail, which are used to fix the device within the vas and prevent sperm from traveling between the device and the vasal wall. The IVD is secured with 1-0 nylon suture around the vas at each sulcus. The IVD is designed to block only spermatozoa, although vasal fluid is allowed to flow through two symmetric holes near the head of the device.

Previous studies of IVDs, namely threads, led to vasal dilation, which would allow spermatozoa to pass beyond the device, decreasing contraceptive efficacy.[40] Song's group suggests that because vasal fluid is allowed to pass, there is no intraluminal increase in pressure or resultant luminal dilation that could potentially allow spermatozoa to pass. Despite these encouraging results, further study is needed before such devices are used in the United States.

POSTOPERATIVE CARE

It is the responsibility of surgeons to review proper postoperative care with patients after vasectomy. Although recommendations may vary with individual surgeons, several common instructions are given to patients. Typically, patients are recommended to apply intermittent ice applications to the scrotum for 8 to 12 hours after the procedure to minimize swelling. Athletic support devices may be worn for scrotal support for 48 hours after the surgery. Postoperative pain is a common concern of vasectomy patients. Acetaminophen alone often provides adequate analgesia. Narcotic analgesia may be necessary, however, and often is prescribed. At the authors' institution, patients are instructed to avoid strenuous activity for 1 week after the procedure. They also are instructed to avoid sexual activity during this period.

POSTVASECTOMY SEMEN ANALSYSIS

Each patient should be counseled that no technique of vasal occlusion is 100% effective. After vasectomy, alternative methods of contraception should be used for 12 weeks as patients are considered fertile until sterility is documented by postvasectomy semen analysis (PVSA). Although no standard protocol for determining sterility exists, semen analysis generally is performed 2 to 3 months after vasectomy. The issue of azoospermia as a required endpoint is controversial. Many investigators advocate performing semen analysis after a minimum of 20 ejaculations post vasectomy in addition to varying time intervals.[2,41] A review of the literature by Griffin and colleagues[42] in 2005 demonstrated evidence that supports a PVSA protocol based on PVSA 3 months and 20 ejaculations after vasectomy. If this PSVA demonstrates azoospermia, patients require no further testing and can be considered sterile. PVSA that show nonmotile sperm at this time, however, require further testing on a monthly basis until azoospermia is documented. If motile sperm are found on the initial PVSA at 3 months post vasectomy, Griffin and colleagues[42] recommend confirming the presence of motile sperm 1 month later before proceeding to revasectomy. Using this protocol, approximately 80% of patients would be cleared after one PVSA.

The need for azoospermia before considering patients sterile, however, recently has been challenged in Europe. Although the finding of motile sperm on PVSA is highly indicative of failed vasectomy, varying amounts of nonmotile sperm are deemed acceptable by many investigators. Limited guidelines in Europe often use from 10,000 to 100,000 nonmotile sperm/mL as appropriately low enough levels of nonmotile sperm to clear patients for unprotected sexual intercourse.[43–47] These recommendations are based on findings that recanalization rates are low when small numbers of nonmotile sperm are found on PVSA.[48,49] Benger and colleagues[48] recommend using a "special clearance" for patients who have persistently low levels of nonmotile sperm as the risk for pregnancy in these patients is estimated to be less than the risk for late recanalization. Surgeons in the United States, however, are subject to a different medicolegal environment than that of their European counterparts and more strict guidelines may be followed.

The use of centrifugation of semen specimens to confirm azoospermia remains controversial yet is practiced in many laboratories in the United States. Steward and colleagues[50] demonstrated that microscopic examination of uncentrifuged semen specimens was highly reliable in identifying samples with 100,000 sperm/mL or more. Given the potential medicolegal implications of not centrifuging specimens when the option is readily available (such as in the United States), this practice likely will continue to be the gold standard for clearance for the foreseeable future.

SUMMARY

Vasectomy remains a safe and effective method of contraception for men. Many variations in surgical technique currently are used by surgeons in the United States, each with its own benefits and drawbacks. Regardless of the surgical method used, the most important factor for successful vasectomy remains the experience and skill of the surgeon. The amount of evidence-based literature on the rationale for the different techniques for vasectomy remains limited. Careful study and innovation of vasectomy techniques will ensure that the most commonly performed urologic surgical procedure remain an excellent form of contraception in the future.

REFERENCES

1. Barone MA, et al. Vasectomy in the United States, 2002. J Urol 2006;176(1):232–6 [discussion: 236].
2. Schwingl PJ, Guess HA. Safety and effectiveness of vasectomy. Fertil Steril 2000;73(5):923–36.
3. Potts JM, et al. Patient characteristics associated with vasectomy reversal. J Urol 1999;161(6):1835–9.
4. Dassow P, Bennett JM. Vasectomy: an update. Am Fam Physician 2006;74(12):2069–74.
5. Sharlip ID. What is the best pregnancy rate that may be expected from vasectomy reversal? J Urol 1993;149(6):1469–71.
6. Goldstein M. Vasectomy reversal. Compr Ther 1993;19(1):37–41.
7. Caesar RE, Kaplan GW. Incidence of the bell-clapper deformity in an autopsy series. Urology 1994;44(1):114–6.
8. Brooks JD. Anatomy of the lower urinary tract and male genitalia. In: Wein AJ, editor. Campell-Walsh urology. 9th edition. Philadelphia: Saunders; 2007. p. 38–77.
9. Kiddoo DA, Wollin TA, Mador DR. A population based assessment of complications following outpatient hydrocelectomy and spermatocelectomy. J Urol 2004;171(2 Pt 1):746–8.
10. Christensen P, et al. [Vasectomy. A prospective, randomized trial of vasectomy with bilateral incision versus the Li vasectomy]. Ugeskr Laeger 2002;164(18):2390–4 [in Danish].
11. Sokal D, et al. A comparative study of the no scalpel and standard incision approaches to vasectomy in 5 countries. The Male Sterilization Investigator Team. J Urol 1999;162(5):1621–5.
12. Cook LA, et al. Scalpel versus no-scalpel incision for vasectomy. Cochrane Database Syst Rev 2007;(2): CD004112.
13. Wolf JS Jr, et al. Best practice policy statement on urologic surgery antimicrobial prophylaxis. J Urol 2008;179(4):1379–90.
14. Wilson W, et al. Prevention of infective endocarditis: guidelines from the American Heart Association: a guideline from the American Heart Association Rheumatic Fever, Endocarditis and Kawasaki Disease Committee, Council on Cardiovascular Disease in the Young, and the Council on Clinical

Cardiology, Council on Cardiovascular Surgery and Anesthesia, and the Quality of Care and Outcomes Research Interdisciplinary Working Group. J Am Dent Assoc 2008;139(Suppl):3S–24S.

15. Holton PD, Leveille RJ, Patzakis MJ, et al. Antibiotic prophylaxis for urological patients with total joint replacements. J Urol 2003;169(5):1796–7.

16. Berry AR, Watt B, Goldacre MJ, et al. A comparison of the use of povidone-iodine and chlorhexidine in the prophylaxis of post-operative wound infection. J Hosp Infect 1982;3(1):55–63.

17. Cooper TP. Use of EMLA cream with vasectomy. Urology 2002;60(1):135–7.

18. Khan AB, Conn IG. Use of EMLA during local anaesthetic vasectomy. Br J Urol 1995;75(5):671.

19. Thomas AA, et al. Topical anesthesia with EMLA does not decrease pain during vasectomy. J Urol 2008;180(1):271–3.

20. Sandlow JI, Winfield HN, Goldstein M. Surgery of the scrotum and seminal vesicles. In: Wein AJ, editor. Campell-Walsh urology. 9th edition. Philadelphia: Saunders; 2007. p. 1098–103.

21. Weiss RS, Li PS. No-needle jet anesthetic technique for no-scalpel vasectomy. J Urol 2005;173(5):1677–80.

22. Li PS, et al. External spermatic sheath injection for vasal nerve block. Urology 1992;39(2):173–6.

23. Li SQ, et al. The no-scalpel vasectomy. J Urol 1991;145(2):341–4.

24. Monoski MA, et al. No-scalpel, no-needle vasectomy. Urology 2006;68(1):9–14.

25. Sokal DC. Recent research on vasectomy techniques. Asian J Androl 2003;5(3):227–30.

26. Jones JS. Percutaneous vasectomy: a simple modification eliminates the steep learning curve of no-scalpel vasectomy. J Urol 2003;169(4):1434–6.

27. Cook LA, et al. Vasectomy occlusion techniques for male sterilization. Cochrane Database Syst Rev 2007;(2):CD003991.

28. Labrecque M, Hoang DQ, Turcot L. Association between the length of the vas deferens excised during vasectomy and the risk of postvasectomy recanalization. Fertil Steril 2003;79(4):1003–7.

29. Labrecque M, et al. Vasectomy surgical techniques in South and South East Asia. BMC Urol 2005;5:10.

30. Gupta AS, Kothari LK, Devpura TP. Vas occlusion by tantalum clips and its comparison with conventional vasectomy in man: reliability, reversibility, and complications. Fertil Steril 1977;28(10):1086–9.

31. Labrecque M, et al. Vasectomy surgical techniques: a systematic review. BMC Med 2004;2:21.

32. Sokal D, et al. Vasectomy by ligation and excision, with or without fascial interposition: a randomized controlled trial [ISRCTN77781689]. BMC Med 2004;2:6.

33. Sokal D, et al. A comparison of vas occlusion techniques: cautery more effective than ligation and excision with fascial interposition. BMC Urol 2004;4(1):12.

34. Barone MA, editor. No-scalpel vasectomy: an illustrated guide for surgeons. 3rd edition. New York: Engender Health; 2003. p. 49.

35. Haws JM, et al. Clinical aspects of vasectomies performed in the United States in 1995. Urology 1998;52(4):685–91.

36. Schmidt SS, Minckler TM. The vas after vasectomy: comparison of cauterization methods. Urology 1992;40(5):468–70.

37. Howards SS, Jessee S, Johnson A. Micropuncture and microanalytic studies of the effect of vasectomy on the rat testis and epididymis. Fertil Steril 1975;26(1):20–7.

38. Silber SJ. Vasectomy reversal. N Engl J Med 1977;296(15):886–7.

39. Song L, et al. A phase II randomized controlled trial of a novel male contraception, an intra-vas device. Int J Androl 2006;29(4):489–95.

40. Lee HY. Experimental studies on reversible vas occlusion by intravasal thread. Fertil Steril 1969;20(5):735–44.

41. Barone MA, et al. A prospective study of time and number of ejaculations to azoospermia after vasectomy by ligation and excision. J Urol 2003;170(3):892–6.

42. Griffin T, et al. How little is enough? The evidence for post-vasectomy testing. J Urol 2005;174(1):29–36.

43. Katsoulis IE, Walker SR. Vasectomy management in Morecambe Bay NHS Trust. Ann R Coll Surg Engl 2005;87(2):131–5.

44. Dohle GR, et al. [Revised guideline 'Vasectomy' from the Dutch Urological Association]. Ned Tijdschr Geneeskd 2005;149(49):2728–31 [in Dutch].

45. Sivardeen KA, Budhoo M. Post vasectomy analysis: call for a uniform evidence-based protocol. Ann R Coll Surg Engl 2001;83(3):177–9.

46. Philp T, Guillebaud J, Budd D. Complications of vasectomy: review of 16,000 patients. Br J Urol 1984;56(6):745–8.

47. Hancock P, McLaughlin E. British Andrology Society guidelines for the assessment of post vasectomy semen samples (2002). J Clin Pathol 2002;55(11):812–6.

48. Benger JR, Swami SK, Gingell JC. Persistent spermatozoa after vasectomy: a survey of British urologists. Br J Urol 1995;76(3):376–9.

49. De Knijff DW, et al. Persistence or reappearance of nonmotile sperm after vasectomy: does it have clinical consequences? Fertil Steril 1997;67(2):332–5.

50. Steward B, Hays M, Sokal D. Diagnostic accuracy of an initial azoospermic reading compared with results of post-centrifugation semen analysis after vasectomy. J Urol 2008;180(5):2119–23.

Effectiveness of Vasectomy Techniques

David C. Sokal, MD[a],*, Michel Labrecque, MD, PhD[b]

KEYWORDS
- Vasectomy methods • Contraception • Recanalization
- Pregnancy • Semen analysis • Review

Modern vasectomy techniques were developed as a component of family planning services in the 1960s and 1970s. Since then, vasectomy has been used as a contraceptive method by millions of couples[1] (see articles by Sheynkin and by Pile and Barone elsewhere in this issue). The procedure is performed in two distinct steps (or three steps if the administration of anesthesia is included as the first step). The first step is the approach to the vas (ie, penetrating the skin and bringing a loop of the vas outside of the scrotum). The second step, which determines contraceptive effectiveness, is to occlude the vas. Many techniques for approaching and occluding the vas have been suggested over the years (see the articles by Sheynkin and by Art and Nangia elsewhere in this issue), and surgeons in the United States and around the world use a wide variety of techniques. This article presents the current knowledge on the effectiveness of the most commonly used vasectomy techniques. To understand vasectomy effectiveness, it is necessary to briefly review the definition and measurement of vasectomy outcomes.

DEFINITION AND MEASUREMENT OF VASECTOMY OUTCOMES

Vasectomy effectiveness may be defined by the absence or occurrence of pregnancy (contraceptive effectiveness) or by the results of semen analyses (occlusive effectiveness).

Contraceptive Effectiveness

Data on pregnancy outcomes have been gathered from two general settings: clinic-based studies and population-based studies. Most published data come from clinical series and family planning clinics. A few reports have provided follow-up data from large clinical series to estimate long-term failure risks.[2–4] Clinic-based studies may underestimate pregnancy rates because of at least three limitations:

- If a pregnancy occurs 1 or more years after a vasectomy, some men may not return to the clinic where they had the vasectomy performed.
- Some women might have an abortion and not inform their partners of a pregnancy because of concerns about marital stability.
- Physicians who have more vasectomy failures are less likely to publish their data.

Only a few population-based studies on the risk for pregnancy in couples relying on vasectomy for family planning have been published. Three studies from outside the United States[5–7] have reported high pregnancy rates (between 3% and

---

This work was partially supported by Family Health International (FHI) with funds from the US Agency for International Development (USAID), Cooperative Agreement GPO-A-00-05-00022-00 (Sokal), and the Fonds de la recherche en santé du Québec (Labrecque). The views expressed in this article are those of the authors and do not necessarily reflect those of FHI, USAID, or Laval University.
a Behavioral and Biomedical Research Department, Family Health International, PO Box 13950, Research Triangle Park, NC 27709, USA
b Département de médecine familiale et de médecine d'urgence, Université Laval, Centre de recherche du CHUQ, D6-728, Hôpital Saint-François d'Assise, CHUQ, 10 rue de l'Espinay, Québec, Québec, Canada
* Corresponding author. Family Health International, 2224 East NC Highway 54, Durham, NC 27713.
E-mail address: dsokal@fhi.org (D.C. Sokal).

Urol Clin N Am 36 (2009) 317–329
doi:10.1016/j.ucl.2009.05.008

9%) 3 to 5 years after vasectomy. These studies are discussed in more detail later.

The risk for pregnancy associated with vasectomy in the United States seems to be relatively low. In a study based on the National Survey of Family Growth,[8] failure risks for vasectomy (and tubal occlusion) were not estimated because "accidental pregnancy is rare with these methods." Based on a survey of US urologists, Deneux-Tharaux and colleagues[9] estimated the risk for pregnancy to be 1 per 1000 procedures, with approximately half of the pregnancies occurring within the first 3 months post vasectomy. Urologists who did more than 50 procedures per year had a lower risk for failures, but no associations were seen between the risk for pregnancy and particular vasectomy techniques. The relatively low risk for pregnancy in the United States may be explained by surgeons' typical use of a combination of vas occlusion techniques.[10] Another US study,[11] however, based on a telephone interview of 540 women whose partners had had a vasectomy, found higher pregnancy rates of 7.4 per 1000 procedures (95% CI, 0.2, 14.6) 1 year after vasectomy and 11.3 per 1000 procedures (95% CI, 2.3, 20.3) up to 5 years after vasectomy.

Although pregnancy prevention is the primary goal, it would be difficult to conduct a prospective study of different vasectomy techniques with pregnancy as the main endpoint. Therefore, prospective studies of the success rates of different vasectomy techniques are based on semen analysis data (ie, occlusive effectiveness) rather than pregnancy rates.

Occlusive Effectiveness

In clinical practice and in most research settings, vasectomy outcomes are defined by the results of one or more semen analyses. In brief, vasectomy success is defined as at least one semen analysis showing no sperm (azoospermia). If only a few nonmotile sperm are observed, most clinicians give a "cautious assurance of success." The presence of any motile sperm indicates a possible vasectomy failure and a risk for pregnancy.

Postvasectomy semen analysis

Various strategies for timing and interpreting the results of postvasectomy semen analysis (PVSA) have been proposed.[12,13] The first PVSA usually is recommended at approximately 12 weeks,[12] or at least 8 weeks after vasectomy.[14] Some practitioners recommend starting as soon as 3 to 4 weeks,[15] and others suggest waiting until 16 weeks.[16] Reflecting the various

recommendations, clinical practice in the United States is extremely diverse.[10]

The rationale for an early test is that if a surgeon's vas occlusion technique is reliable, then only small numbers of nonmotile sperm should be present by 3 to 4 weeks post vasectomy, and the ability of such residual sperm to fertilize an ovum is doubtful.[17–19] Jouannet and David wrote, "Motile spermatozoa were never observed after the 15th day following vasectomy. The reappearance of motile spermatozoa after that time was an almost certain sign of a defect in the vas block or of recanalization of the vas deferens."[17]

The reason that has been proposed for later testing, at 16 weeks, is to allow time for men who have slow sperm clearance to reach azoospermia and avoid the need for a second PVSA.

There is wide variation among clinicians in the number of PVSA deemed necessary to confirm vas occlusion.[10,20] Based on most recent evidence, only one completely azoospermic semen specimen is sufficient to confirm occlusion.[12] Moreover, most experts classify probable success and provide "special clearance" or "cautious assurance of success" when only small numbers of nonmotile sperm are present.[12,13,21,22] The initial article defining special clearance suggested a nonmotile sperm cutoff level of 10,000/mL,[21] but a description of the laboratory methods used by the investigators was never published. More recently, investigators,[23,24] and guidelines from the British Andrology Society[16] and the Dutch Urological Association[25] have suggested a nonmotile sperm cutoff level of 100,000/mL.

Readers can find additional information about semen analysis techniques in the World Health Organization's manual for semen analysis,[26] in Mortimer's *Practical Laboratory Andrology*,[27] and in other published articles.[24,28] Although some authorities recommend centrifugation to document azoospermia,[16] a recent article suggests that a careful examination of noncentrifuged specimens may be sufficient.[24] Mortimer provides detailed instructions on how to estimate sperm concentration in uncentrifuged wet preparations based on the volume of the drop of semen, the coverslip size, and the particular microscope's field of view. (A calculation that was cited occasionally in the older literature was that 1 sperm/high power field [hpf] of a wet preparation is equal to 1 million sperm/mL. With modern, wide-field microscopes, however, the field of vision is larger and that estimate is probably no longer valid in most laboratories. With modern microscopes, and a small, 10-μL drop of liquefied semen under a 22-mm coverslip, 1 sperm/hpf = approximately

250,000 sperm/mL [calculated from data in Mortimer's Table 3.1, page 49, and Appendix II]).

In 2008, the Food and Drug Administration approved the first home test kit, SpermCheck Vasectomy,[29] for men to perform their own PVSA at home. It is similar to a home pregnancy test but uses semen rather than urine. Among 144 postvasectomy semen samples, the test was always positive (100% sensitivity) with sperm counts above 385,000 sperm/mL.[29] At that cutoff, the test should identify most cases of early recanalization, the most common cause of vasectomy failure. Sperm motility cannot be assessed with this test, however, requiring standard semen analysis in case of a positive result.

Recanalization and occlusive outcomes

Postvasectomy recanalization of the vas may be defined most simply as the growth of new connections between the proximal and distal cut ends of the vas, permitting the passage of sperm (This article uses the term *recanalization* to refer to spontaneous postvasectomy recanalization, but in some countries other than the United States, recanalization may be used to refer to vasectomy reversal surgery [ie, vasovasostomy and related procedures]). The pathophysiology of recanalization remains unclear, however. Current limited understanding is based mainly on histopathologic studies that have been conducted on specimens collected from men undergoing repeat vasectomy or vasovasostomy.[30–35] Various tissues and cells, including connective tissue, spermatozoa, blood cells, smooth muscle tissue, and epithelial cells, are involved in a granulomatous reaction that bridges the gap between the cut ends of the vas deferens. Epithelial-lined microtubules proliferate through the granulomatous tissue, producing a fistula that allows the passage of sperm.

Recanalizations usually are classified as early or late. Early recanalization can be diagnosed when a man shows motile sperm on a routine PVSA at 8 to 12 weeks and may be suspected if a man shows more than 1 million nonmotile sperm/mL at that time. A late recanalization is one that occurs after a man has been declared sterile. Late recanalizations are relatively rare and usually are identified after the occurrence of a pregnancy.

Before recent work by Family Health International and EngenderHealth, only a few others had published data using serial semen analyses to document early recanalizations.[36,37] By analyzing serial samples from 400 vasectomy cases, Marshall and Lyon[36] reported eight men who had a transient re-appearance of sperm. Similarly, Esho and coworkers[37] reported six cases of early recanalization. In four of the cases of early recanalization with repeat vasectomies, they reported seeing recanalization channels by histopathology and by radiographic study of the excised vas segments.

A decade of research led by Family Health International and EngenderHealth, with funding from the US Agency for International Development and assistance from many collaborators, has helped further understanding of the frequency of early and transient recanalizations, especially when ligation and excision are used for vas occlusion. In three prospective clinical trials, the investigators collected multiple semen samples beginning as early as 2 weeks post vasectomy, including data from more than 1400 men.[38–41] Early recanalizations were more common than generally realized, as high as 25% with simple ligation and excision of a short vas segment. Approximately half of the recanalizations were subclinical or transient.

Based on the authors' work, possible vasectomy outcomes have been identified and classified into two categories, success or failure (**Table 1**). **Figs. 1** and **2** illustrate the semen clearance patterns associated with these outcomes, except for late recanalizations. Each line in the figures shows PVSA results for one man, with semen analyses done every 2 weeks.[41]

Occlusive outcomes without recanalization Cases 1 to 3 are successes and case 4 is a failure (see **Fig. 1**). Cases 1 and 2 show rapid achievement of azoospermia. In case 3, the sperm concentration rapidly drops below 1 million sperm/mL, but the decrease to azoospermia is much slower. This may be explained by individual differences in anatomy or sperm flow or by age. In some men, residual nonmotile sperm may take longer to dislodge from the complex folds of the ampullary region of the vas or from the passages of the seminal vesicles.[42] Older men commonly take longer to reach azoospermia than younger men.[39,43] In cases 1 to 3, no motile sperm were seen after the 2-week semen analysis.

Case 4 was presumed a surgical error (ie, one vas was not occluded). The sperm concentration never dropped, and all samples showed motile sperm. Such technical failures are so rare among experienced surgeons that it is difficult to estimate their frequency. A surgeon occasionally may operate twice on the same vas, thus leaving one vas unoccluded. More rarely, an anatomic variation, such as a duplicate vas deferens, may lead to a technical failure. Given the usual timing of the first semen analysis in clinical settings, it may not be possible to tell the difference between a technical/surgical failure and an early recanalization based solely on the semen analysis results.

| Table 1 |
Possible postvasectomy occlusive outcomes
Success
"Normal" success (see **Fig. 1**, cases 1 to 3)
Transient early recanalization
Success before first PVSA (subclinical recanalization) (see **Fig. 2**, cases 5 and 6)
Success after first PVSA (delayed success) (see **Fig. 2**, case 7)
Failure
Technical/surgical error (see **Fig. 1**, case 4)
Persistent early recanalization (see **Fig. 2**, case 8)
Late failure
Persistent late recanalization
Transient late recanalization

Occlusive outcomes with recanalization **Fig. 2** shows the PVSA results of four men who had presumed recanalization: three men had transient recanalization, with subsequent scarring of the vas lumen resulting in vasectomy success, and one man had persistent recanalization, a vasectomy failure. The recanalizations in cases 5 and 6 probably would not be recognized by a surgeon in the usual clinical setting, because the first PVSA is commonly done at 12 weeks, when both men would be azoospermic or close to azoospermic. Cases 5 and 6 probably would have been considered normal successful vasectomies (ie, subclinical recanalization).

Case 7 would be identified at his first PVSA as a possible failure, but subsequent PVSA showed that he reached success (albeit delayed) after a transient recanalization. Delayed success occurs by 6 months in approximately 50% of men who have motile sperm at the time of their first PVSA and are considered to have an early recanalization.[44]

Case 8 was azoospermic at 2 weeks, but the sperm concentration rapidly returned to normal levels with motile sperm and persisted. This is a persistent early recanalization and was considered a vasectomy failure at 24 weeks. This probably is the most common type of failure that surgeons see. In the research context, the authors

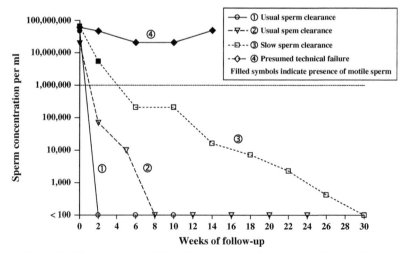

Fig. 1. Semen analysis charts of four men who did not have presumed early recanalization. Sperm concentration is illustrated on a logarithmic scale. Because a logarithmic scale has no true zero, <100 on the graph was used to indicate azoospermia. The dotted line indicates low sperm cutoff (1,000,000 sperm/mL) according to reviewers' consensus. For case 2, prevasectomy sperm concentrations were not available. A count of 20,000,000 sperm/mL with presence of motile sperm was assumed. (*From* Labrecque M, Hays M, Chen-Mok M, et al. Frequency and patterns of early recanalization after vasectomy. BMC Urol 2006;6:25; under a Creative Commons license, http://creativecommons.org/licenses/by/2.0/; with permission.)

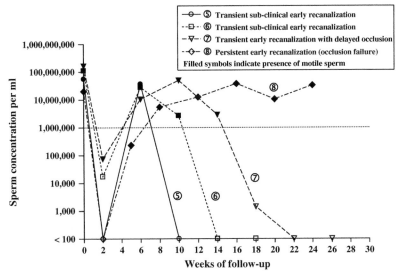

Fig. 2. Semen analysis charts of four men who had presumed early recanalization. Sperm concentration is illustrated on a logarithmic scale. Because a logarithmic scale has no true zero, <100 on the graph was used to indicate azoospermia. The dotted line indicates low sperm cutoff (1,000,000 sperm/mL) according to reviewers' consensus. For case 8, prevasectomy sperm concentrations were not available. A count of 20,000,000 sperm/mL with presence of motile sperm was assumed. (*From* Labrecque M, Hays M, Chen-Mok M, et al. Frequency and patterns of early recanalization after vasectomy. BMC Urol 2006;6:25; under a Creative Commons license, http://creativecommons.org/licenses/by/2.0/; with permission.)

defined success and failure by a man's status at 6 months, so case 8 was considered a vasectomy failure. In clinical practice, however, many surgeons might follow such a case with monthly semen analyses for more than 6 months before doing a repeat vasectomy. Such cases eventually may show a decline to azoospermia and become delayed successes. In a study that followed 36 such men,[39] 10 of them eventually achieved vasectomy success by 42 weeks post vasectomy.

Late recanalization Although a few surgeons[37] have suggested that men return for annual PVSA to identify failures due to late recanalization, subsequent research has shown that the risk for late failure after documented azoospermia is too low to justify routine annual testing. Philp and colleagues[2] and Davies and colleagues[21] at the Elliot-Smith Clinic, have provided key data on long-term outcomes. Philp and colleagues reported long-term follow-up data on 14,047 men who had confirmed azoospermia on two rounds of PVSA and estimated that the risk for pregnancy after azoospermia was approximately 1 in 2000 men. Davies and colleagues reported long-term follow-up data on 151 men at the clinic who had been given "special clearance" based on the continued presence of small numbers of nonmotile sperm. These men were older than average patients at the clinic, with age perhaps contributing to a slower clearance of sperm. Upon semen analysis at later follow-up, at

least three or more years post vasectomy, all but one of the men were azoospermic and none of their partners had become pregnant. A single man still had small numbers of sperm present in his semen, estimated at less than 5000/mL.

Data on men requesting vasectomy reversal from infertility clinics show that even many years after vasectomy, 10% to 20% of men have small numbers of nonmotile sperm that can be detected by careful examination after centrifugation.[45,46] This suggests another reason not to recommend annual PVSA, because results could lead to repeat vasectomies in men who have very low sperm counts and a remote risk for pregnancy.

If a postvasectomy pregnancy does occur, physicians should assume that the pregnancy is due to recanalization, even if the results of a semen analysis are negative. Transient late recanalizations resulting in pregnancy—with negative semen samples after diagnosis of the pregnancy—have been well documented by genetic testing.[47–49] Physicians should not suggest that a man's spouse may have had another sexual partner unless genetic testing has been performed to rule out fatherhood by the vasectomized man.

EFFECTIVENESS OF VASECTOMY OCCLUSION TECHNIQUES

Many vasectomy occlusion techniques have been developed over the years, and these techniques continue to evolve (see the articles by Sheynkin and by Art and Nangia elsewhere in this issue). The authors have reviewed the effectiveness of the vas occlusion techniques that are most commonly used in the United States.[10]

Most physicians use a combination of these techniques (some investigators do not classify the last four techniques as methods of vas occlusion):

- Ligation
- Cautery (intraluminal)
- Clips
- Excision of a segment of the vas
- Fascial interposition (FI)
- Fold back one or two vasal ends
- Open-ended vasectomy (testicular end)

Details on how each of these common techniques is performed are provided (see the article by Art and Nangia elsewhere in this issue). Techniques for approaching the vas (such as the no-scalpel technique) have no influence on vasectomy effectiveness and are not considered in this article.

There are many challenges to interpreting published data on the effectiveness of vasectomy techniques, including incomplete follow-up (discussed previously). Another challenge is that few studies have been performed on any particular technique, and those studies that have been performed primarily are retrospective reviews of individual physicians' experiences. Moreover, study details often are lacking; definitions of techniques and outcomes vary; failure is based mostly on semen analysis but without defining the laboratory methods or criteria explicitly; and follow-up data often are relatively short-term and unsystematic.

The following summaries of vasectomy occlusion technique effectiveness are based on a systematic review of comparative studies of vasectomy techniques published in 2004 by Labrecque and colleagues[50] and on a Cochrane review of randomized clinical trials updated in 2007.[51] To find more recent comparative studies to include in this article, the authors searched MEDLINE for articles published between June 2003 and February 2009, using the keywords, "vasectomy" and "humans"; 349 articles were identified, but only one new study compared two vasectomy occlusion techniques.[52]

In what follows, level A evidence refers to randomized controlled trials or meta-analyses, and level B evidence refers to other types of studies.

Ligation and Excision

Ligation and excision of the vas is the most common method of vas occlusion in developing countries,[6,44] although the data documenting this are limited. Suture material or metal clips can be used to ligate the vas. In the United States, only approximately 6.9% of surgeons use simple ligation and excision with suture material and 6.8% use simple ligation and excision with metal clips (based on data from Barone and colleagues: [16.9% of surgeons use ligation alone] × [100 − 59.3% of those surgeons not using FI] = 6.9% for suture ligation alone; [8.8% × (100 − 22.2%)] = 6.8% for clip ligation alone).[10] Some practitioners who use clips, however, report using more than one clip on each end of each vas. Most surgeons excise a vas segment from between the ligatures—usually between 0.5 cm and 4 cm but most commonly approximately 1 cm.

How the vas is ligated may affect the likelihood of failure. Applying too much pressure when putting sutures or clips on the vas deferens, which is a smooth muscle, is common. Too tight a ligature creates ischemia and eventually causes necrosis and sloughing of the ligated stump, leading to recanalization. Alternatively, if the ligature is too loose, occlusion will fail. For these reasons, many investigators have recommended not putting any sutures or clips on the vas deferens.[4,53,54]

The risk for vasectomy failure with this technique traditionally has been considered to be high, between 1% and 5%.[55] Recent, more rigorous studies, however, have shown that the risk could be much higher, ranging from 8% to 13% based on data from semen analyses.[38,39,56] The risk for recanalization is even higher. In the authors' study assessing the frequency and patterns of recanalization, the risks for vasectomy failure and early recanalization were estimated to be 13% and 25%, respectively, among 416 men who provided serial postvasectomy semen samples up to 6 months after vasectomy (**Table 2**).[41]

The risk for contraceptive failure also may be high, as illustrated in studies in which most vasectomies were done by simple ligation and excision.[44] In a population-based cross-sectional study of family planning conducted in China, the cumulative pregnancy rate among 1555 couples relying on vasectomy was 9.5% at 5 years.[5] A population-based study of 1052 men in Nepal[6] estimated a cumulative pregnancy rate of 4.2% at 3 years or 3% at 3 years excluding pregnancies occurring within the first 3 months post vasectomy. The Nepal study is unique among population-based studies in that Nazerali and colleagues (1) collected semen samples and (2) they were able to obtain limited data on surgical techniques. A similar pregnancy rate (4.1%) was found in Vietnam after more than 5 years of follow-up.[7] Finally, in a retrospective clinic-based

Table 2
Risk for occlusive failure and early recanalization according to vasectomy occlusion techniques

Outcomes	Ligation and Excision		Cautery	
	FI−	FI+	FI−	FI+
	N = 414	n = 410	n = 197	n = 192
Occlusive failure (%)[a]	13	5	1	0.5[b]
Recanalization (%)	25	10	9	0

Abbreviations: FI−, without FI; FI+, with FI.
[a] Occlusive failure was defined as 10 million sperm/mL at 12 weeks or later.
[b] Including one technically failed vasectomy.

study in India, 3% to 5% of couples using vasectomy had a pregnancy after 5 years.[57]

Metal clips do not seem to increase effectiveness when compared with any of the suture materials used in the few comparative studies available.[50] A recently published retrospective comparative case series showed that ligating the vas with Vicryl results in a significantly higher failure rate in achieving azoospermia (10.1% of 1088 men) than does ligating with chromic catgut (3.5% of 1038 men).[52]

Failure is rare when a 4-cm or larger vas segment is excised.[58–62] Excising such a long segment, however, requires extensive dissection of the vas and may be associated with a higher risk for surgical complications. Moreover, it may preclude successful vasovasostomy. Excising a longer segment within the range of 0.5 cm to 2 cm is not associated with a lower risk for failure.[63]

VasClip, which is a single clip system that does not require cutting the vas, had been proposed as an alternative occlusion method. The risk for failure for VasClip seems similar or higher than that for simple ligation and excision, based on two published reports.[64,65] The VasClip company has apparently stopped marketing the device due to the high failure rate. (The VasClip Web site, vasclip.com, is no longer active, and the company's phone number is no longer in service.)

In brief, simple ligation and excision (with no other techniques) is associated with a relatively high risk for failure and no longer recommended.[14,66]

Fascial Interposition

To increase the effectiveness of vasectomy, some physicians have recommended creating a tissue barrier between the severed ends of the vas by pulling the internal spermatic fascia (the sheath covering the vas deferens) over one of the vas stumps. This technique is named fascial interposition (FI). The fascia can be sealed over the testicular or the prostatic end using suture materiel or a metal clip.

Five studies comparing vas occlusion techniques with FI versus without FI were reported in a systematic review published in 2004.[50] **Table 3** presents the risk for occlusive failure reported in these five studies.[39,67–71] Although the specific occlusion techniques differed among the studies, all used some form of ligation and excision, with the exception of one study in which the vas was only transected.[68] Only three studies clearly described how the FI was performed. The fascia was sealed over the prostatic end in one study[67] and over the testicular end in the other two.[39,69] Although the risk for failure varied largely from one study to the next, all of the studies showed fewer failures with FI.

Mainly based on the single large randomized trial by Sokal and colleagues,[39] there is good evidence that FI reduces the risk for occlusive failure of vasectomy performed with ligation and excision. Even in this study, however, the risk for failure (5%) and of presumed early recanalization (10%) were unacceptably high (see **Table 2**).

Cautery (Thermal or Electrical)

Intraluminal thermal (hot-wire) or electrical cautery of the vas lumen has been advocated as an effective vas occlusion technique, used alone or combined with FI.

Cautery without fascial interposition
Ligation and excision with or without FI and cautery without FI were compared in six studies.[41,69–74] Results have not been not consistent (**Table 4**). The largest study, which was performed in the United Kingdom with electrical cautery, did not find any difference between the techniques.[74] Three of the studies found better results with ligation and excision,[69,72,73] and two found better results with cautery.[70,71,75] It is thus difficult to draw definitive conclusions on the effectiveness

Table 3
Risk for occlusive failure in studies comparing vasectomy performed with simple ligation and excision versus ligation and excision combined with fascial interposition

Study	Study Design	Sample Size		Side of Fascial Interposition	Occlusive Failure (%)[a]	
		LE	LE + FI		LE	LE + FI
Schmidt, 1973	III	150	135	Prostatic	3.3	0
Rhodes, 1980	III	28	12	Unspecified	21.4	16.7
Li, 1994	II	183	186	Testicular	7.5	0.6
De los Rios, 1994 and 2003	III	550	302	Unspecified	29.1	2.6
Sokal 2003	I	422	419	Testicular	12.7	5.9

Study design. I: randomized clinical trial or quasirandomized clinical trial. II: nonrandomized parallel group trial, before-and-after trial (prospective experimental study of different techniques conducted over different time periods), or prospective cohort study. III: case-control study, retrospective cohort study, or retrospective case series with historical or concurrent controls.

Abbreviations: FI, fascial interposition; LE, ligation and excision.

[a] Definitions of occlusive failure are not uniform across studies.

of cautery, especially because none of these studies provide level A evidence (see **Table 4**).

Cautery with fascial interposition

Seven studies have compared the risk for occlusive failure with ligation and excision with or without FI versus cautery with FI (**Table 5**).[4,41,56,67,76–82] Although none of the studies provides level A evidence, all seven studies found a small risk for occlusive failure with cautery combined with FI (0.5% or less in six of the seven

studies). In all seven studies, the risk for occlusive failure was much lower for cautery than for ligation and excision.

The authors did not find any studies comparing cautery without FI and cautery with FI. The risk for occlusive failure was lower, however, on average, in the seven studies of cautery with FI than in the five studies of cautery without FI (see **Tables 4** and **5**). In addition, in the authors and colleagues' study of frequency and patterns of recanalization,[41] no recanalization was observed

Table 4
Risk for occlusive failure in studies comparing vasectomy performed with ligation and excision combined or not with fascial interposition and simple cautery

Study	Study Design	Sample Size		Type of Cautery	Occlusive Failures (%)[a]	
		LE/LE + FI	C		LE/LE + FI	C
Bangstrup, 1977	II	324	254	Electrical	2.7	3.5
Shapiro, 1979	II	262	148	Thermal	0.4	3.1
Philp, 1984	III	4500	12,300	Electrical	0.5	0.3
Li, 1994	II	427/186	442	Electrical	1.4/0.6	4.8
De Los Rios, 1994 and 2003	III	550/302	131	Thermal	29.1/2.6	1.2
Labrecque, 2006[b]	II	414/410	197	Electrical	12.7/4.9	1.0

Study design. I: randomized clinical trial or quasirandomized clinical trial. II: nonrandomized parallel group trial, before-and-after trial (prospective experimental study of different techniques conducted over different time periods), or prospective cohort study. III: case-control study, retrospective cohort study, or retrospective case series with historical or concurrent controls.

Abbreviations: C, cautery; FI, fascial interposition; LE, ligation and excision.

[a] Definitions of occlusive failure are not uniform across studies.

[b] Combines data from two studies. Original data were reported by Sokal and colleagues[39] and Barone and colleagues.[40]

Table 5
Risk for occlusive failure in studies comparing vasectomy performed with ligation and excision combined or not with fascial interposition and cautery combined with fascial interposition

| Study | Study Design | Sample Size | | Type of Cautery | Occlusive Failures (%)[a] | |
		LE/LE + FI	C + FI		LE/LE + FI	C + FI
Moss, 1972, 1976, and 1992	III	551	6184	Thermal	0.5	0.03
Schmidt, 1973, 1978, and 1995	III	150/135	6248	Thermal	3.3	0
Esho, 1978	III	497	820	Electrical	6.5	0.5
Simcock, 1978	III	790	1649	Electrical	1.4	0.3
Labrecque, 1998	III	545	322	Thermal	2.8	1.2
Labrecque, 2002	II–III	1453	1165	Thermal	8.7	0.3
Labrecque, 2006[b]	II	414/410	192	Thermal	12.7/4.9	0.5

Study design. I: randomized clinical trial or quasirandomized clinical trial. II: nonrandomized parallel group trial, before-and-after trial (prospective experimental study of different techniques conducted over different time periods), or prospective cohort study. III: case-control study, retrospective cohort study, or retrospective case series with historical or concurrent controls.

Abbreviations: C, cautery; FI, fascial interposition; LE, ligation and excision.

[a] Definitions of occlusive failure are not uniform across studies.

[b] Combines data from two studies. Original data were reported by Sokal and colleagues[39] and Barone and colleagues.[40]

in patients who had their vasectomy performed with intraluminal cautery combined with FI (see **Table 2**).

Based on these comparative studies, there are no apparent differences in the risks for failure for thermal and electrical intraluminal cautery. Only one clinical study actually compared the two types of cautery. The difference in the risk for occlusive failure was not statistically significant (3.1% for thermal cautery and 6.1% for electrical cautery).[69] When the sealing of the vas was assessed by the number of cases of vasitis nodosa and spermatic granuloma at the time of vasectomy reversal, however, thermal cautery showed better results than electrical cautery.[83]

In 2002, Marie Stopes International published a case series of 45,123 men who were vasectomized using an electrocautery technique without cutting the vas.[84] Electrocautery was used to access the vas (a no-scalpel approach) and to destroy the vas almost completely for a distance of 2 to 3 cm, leaving intact only a thin portion of the posterior wall of the vas. The reported failure rate was 0.7%. An attempt to use intraluminal thermal cautery without cutting the vas, however, proved to be associated with a high risk for failure.

In a cohort of the 135 men who provided at least one sample for PVSA, 30% had motile sperm at the time of the first PVSA. The incidence of possible or confirmed occlusive failure in these men was 15%.[85]

Folding Back a Vas Segment

Folding back one or both vas segments on themselves and maintaining them in place with a suture has been advocated to increase vasectomy effectiveness. Five studies have compared vas ligation with folding back and vas ligation (with or without excision) without folding back.[50] Two of the studies found a similar risk for occlusive failure between vas ligation with and without folding back when clips were used in the comparison group.[86,87] Two studies found fewer occlusive failures with folding back,[70,71,81] and one found more occlusive and contraceptive failures with folding back.[69] One population-based study[6] found fewer failures by a single surgeon who used a fold-back technique compared with others using simple ligation and excision. Considering the overall results of the studies and their methodologic quality, there was no clear advantage of folding back in terms of increasing effectiveness.

Leaving the Testicular End Open (Open-ended Vasectomy)

Leaving the testicular end open has been proposed to decrease the back pressure on the epididymis and reduce the risk for postvasectomy chronic pain. A reduction in damage to the epididymis has been demonstrated in animal models.[88] Based on current clinical evidence, however, no firm conclusions can be made about the potential benefit of the open-ended technique in reducing the risk for postvasectomy chronic pain in humans.[50] Another potential advantage of the open-ended technique is that it might increase the probability of success after vasectomy reversal, but the authors are not aware of any comparative studies measuring this outcome.

A major advantage of using an open-ended vasectomy technique is that it reduces the time to perform the surgical procedure. Some clinicians are reluctant to leave the testicular end open, however, fearing the increased occurrence of sperm granuloma associated with this technique and subsequent pain[78,89] and occlusive failure. Results from studies comparing the open-ended technique to a technique in which the testicular end is closed suggest that the open-ended technique does not increase the risk for chronic pain and occlusive failure when the prostatic end is adequately occluded using FI and cautery (**Table 6**).[56,69,73,78,82,89]

SUMMARY AND RECOMMENDATIONS

In the United States and other high-resource settings, there seem to be fewer vasectomy failures and fewer postvasectomy pregnancies than in low-resource settings. This is probably due mainly to differences in vas occlusion methods and subsequent recanalizations.

Given the number of vasectomy procedures performed annually around the world, there is surprisingly little high-quality evidence on the relative effectiveness of various techniques for vas occlusion. Nonetheless, taking into account the limitations of the available studies, the authors propose the following conclusions and recommendations:

1. Recanalization is the most common reason for vasectomy failure (evidence level B). As a randomized trial to study this outcome does not seem feasible, level B evidence probably will remain the best level of evidence available.
2. Simple ligation and excision, with suture material (evidence level A) or surgical clips (evidence level B), is associated with an unacceptably high risk for failure and should not be used as a vasectomy occlusion technique.
3. Adding FI to ligation and excision significantly reduces the risk for failure (evidence level A).
4. Techniques that include cautery seem to have a lower risk for failure than techniques that do

Table 6
Risk for occlusive failure in studies comparing vasectomy performed with testicular end left open versus close end

| Study | Study Design | Sample Size | | Type of Occlusion on Prostatic End | Occlusive Failures (%)[a] | |
		Open	Close		Open	Close
Goldstein, 1978	III	4	387	TC	50	0.3
Shapiro, 1979	III	23	91	LE or TC	2.1	0
Errey, 1986	III	3867	4330	EC + FI + FB	0.02	0.08
Moss, 1992	III	3103	3081	TC + FI	0.03	0.03
Li, 1994	II	415	2298	LE + FI	4.1	3.1
Labrecque, 1998	III	322	545	TC + FI	1.2	2.8
Labrecque, 2002	II–III	1165	1453	TC + FI	0.3	8.7

Study design. I: randomized clinical trial or quasirandomized clinical trial. II: nonrandomized parallel group trial, before-and-after trial (prospective experimental study of different techniques conducted over different time periods), or prospective cohort study. III: case-control study, retrospective cohort study, or retrospective case series with historical or concurrent controls.

Abbreviations: EC, electrical cautery; FB, folding back; FI, fascial interposition; LE, ligation and excision; TC, thermal cautery.

[a] Definitions of occlusive failure are not uniform across studies.

not include cautery (evidence level B). There is insufficient evidence to recommend a particular standardized cautery technique, but adding FI to cautery seems to be associated with the lowest risk for failure.

5. Open-ended vasectomy does not increase the risk for failure when the prostatic end is adequately closed using FI and cautery (evidence level B).

6. Additional research is needed to a) clarify the importance of including FI with thermal or electrical cautery (the Indian Council of Medical Research is planning to conduct a randomized controlled trial to compare ligation and excision combined with FI [the current government-recommended method in India]; thermal cautery and excision; and thermal cautery and excision combined with FI. In all three groups, surgeons plan to use the no-scalpel vasectomy approach to the vas and to excise approximately 1 cm of the vas); b) document any potential benefits of the open-ended technique; and c) explore new ideas for quicker and easier methods of vas occlusion.

ACKNOWLEDGMENTS

The authors thank their many colleagues and coauthors at FHI, EngenderHealth, and around the world who contributed to the studies reviewed in this article. Also, thanks to Kerry Aradhya for editorial assistance.

REFERENCES

1. EngenderHealth. Contraceptive sterilization: global issues and trends. New York: EngenderHealth; 2002.

2. Philp T, Guillebaud J, Budd D. Late failure of vasectomy after two documented analyses showing azoospermic semen. Br Med J (Clin Res Ed) 1984;289: 77–9.

3. Alderman PM. The lurking sperm. A review of failures in 8879 vasectomies performed by one physician. JAMA 1988;259:3142–4.

4. Schmidt SS. Vasectomy by section, luminal fulguration and fascial interposition: results from 6248 cases. Br J Urol 1995;76:373–4 [discussion: 375].

5. Wang D. Contraceptive failure in China. Contraception 2002;66:173–8.

6. Nazerali H, Thapa S, Hays M, et al. Vasectomy effectiveness in Nepal: a retrospective study. Contraception 2003;67:397–401.

7. Hieu DT, Luong TT, Anh PT, et al. The acceptability, efficacy and safety of quinacrine non-surgical sterilization (QS), tubectomy and vasectomy in 5 provinces in the Red River Delta, Vietnam: a follow-up

8. Fu H, Darroch JE, Haas T, et al. Contraceptive failure rates: new estimates from the 1995 National Survey of Family Growth. Fam Plann Perspect 1999;31:56–63.

9. Deneux-Tharaux C, Kahn E, Nazerali H, et al. Pregnancy rates after vasectomy: a survey of US urologists. Contraception 2004;69:401–6.

10. Barone MA, Hutchinson PL, Johnson CH, et al. Vasectomy in the United States, 2002. J Urol 2006; 176:232–6 [discussion: 236].

11. Jamieson DJ, Costello C, Trussell J, et al. The risk of pregnancy after vasectomy. Obstet Gynecol 2004; 103:848–50.

12. Griffin T, Tooher R, Nowakowski K, et al. How little is enough? The evidence for post-vasectomy testing. J Urol 2005;174:29–36.

13. Labrecque M, Barone MA, Pile J, et al. Re: how little is enough? The evidence for post-vasectomy testing. J Urol 2006;175:791–2 [author reply: 792].

14. Royal College of Obstetricians & Gynaecologists. Male and female sterilization, evidence-based clinical guideline no. 4. London: RCOG Press; 2004.

15. Edwards IS. Earlier testing after vasectomy, based on the absence of motile sperm. Fertil Steril 1993; 59:431–6.

16. Hancock P, McLaughlin E. British Andrology Society guidelines for the assessment of post vasectomy semen samples (2002). J Clin Pathol 2002;55:812–6.

17. Jouannet P, David G. Evolution of the properties of semen immediately following vasectomy. Fertil Steril 1978;29:435–41.

18. Lewis EL, Brazil CK, Overstreet JW. Human sperm function in the ejaculate following vasectomy. Fertil Steril 1984;42:895–8.

19. Richardson DW, Aitken RJ, Loudon NB. The functional competence of human spermatozoa recovered after vasectomy. J Reprod Fertil 1984;70: 575–9.

20. Benger JR, Swami SK, Gingell JC. Persistent spermatozoa after vasectomy: a survey of British urologists. Br J Urol 1995;76:376–9.

21. Davies AH, Sharp RJ, Cranston D, et al. The long-term outcome following "special clearance" after vasectomy. Br J Urol 1990;66:211–2.

22. Sandlow J, Winfield H, Goldstein M. Surgical of the scrotum and seminal vesicles. In: Wein A, Kavoussi L, Novick A, et al. editors. Campbell-Walsh urology. 9th edition. Philadelphia: Saunders; 2006. p. 1098–127.

23. Rajmil O, Fernandez M, Rojas-Cruz C, et al. [Azoospermia should not be given as the result of vasectomy]. Arch Esp Urol 2007;60:55–8 [in Spanish].

24. Steward B, Hays M, Sokal D. Diagnostic accuracy of an initial azoospermic reading compared with results of post-centrifugation semen analysis after vasectomy. J Urol 2008;180:2119–23.

of 15,190 cases. Int J Gynaecol Obstet 2003; 83(Suppl 2):S77–85.

25. Dohle GR, Meuleman EJ, Hoekstra JW, et al. [Revised guideline 'Vasectomy' from the Dutch Urological Association]. Ned Tijdschr Geneeskd 2005;149:2728–31 [in Dutch].

26. World Health Organization. WHO laboratory manual for the examination of human semen and sperm-cervical mucus interaction. 99. Cambridge, England: Cambridge University Press; 1999.

27. Mortimer D. Practical laboratory andrology. New York: Oxford University Press; 1994.

28. Chafer Rudilla M, Navarro Casado L, Belilty Araque M, et al. [Influence of the analytical process in the appearance and disappearance of the spermatozoa after vasectomy]. Actas Urol Esp 2007; 31:270–5 [in Spanish].

29. Klotz KL, Coppola MA, Labrecque M, et al. Clinical and consumer trial performance of a sensitive immunodiagnostic home test that qualitatively detects low concentrations of sperm following vasectomy. J Urol 2008;180:2569–76.

30. Cruickshank B, Eidus L, Barkin M. Regeneration of vas deferens after vasectomy. Urology 1987;30: 137–42 [in Spanish].

31. Hayashi H, Cedenho AP, Sadi A. The mechanism of spontaneous recanalization of human vasectomized ductus deferens. Fertil Steril 1983;40:269–70.

32. Wei C. [Multiple tiny channels, a type of reanastomosis after vasectomy: a pathological study of 38 cases]. Shengzhi Yu Biyun 1987;7:61–2 [in Chinese].

33. Pugh RC, Hanley HG. Spontaneous recanalisation of the divided vas deferens. Br J Urol 1969;41:340–7.

34. Freund MJ, Weidmann JE, Goldstein M, et al. Micro-recanalization after vasectomy in man. J Androl 1989;10:120–32.

35. Schmidt SS, Morris RR. Spermatic granuloma: the complication of vasectomy. Fertil Steril 1973;24: 941–7.

36. Marshall, S., Lyon, R.P. Transient reappearance of sperm after vasectomy. JAMA 1972;219(13):1753–4. 72.

37. Esho JO, Ireland GW, Cass AS. Recanalization following vasectomy. Urology 1974;3:211–4.

38. Barone MA, Nazerali H, Cortes M, et al. A prospective study of time and number of ejaculations to azoospermia after vasectomy by ligation and excision. J Urol 2003;170:892–6.

39. Sokal D, Irsula B, Hays M, et al. Vasectomy by ligation and excision, with or without fascial interposition: a randomized controlled trial. BMC Med 2004;2:6.

40. Barone MA, Irsula B, Chen-Mok M, et al. Effectiveness of vasectomy using cautery. BMC Urol 2004;4:10.

41. Labrecque M, Hays M, Chen-Mok M, et al. Frequency and patterns of early recanalization after vasectomy. BMC Urol 2006;6:25.

42. Mumford SD, Davis JE, Freund M. Considerations in selecting a postvasectomy semen examination regimen. Int Urol Nephrol 1982;14:293–306.

43. Spencer B, Charlesworth D. Factors determining the rate of disappearance of sperm from the ejaculate after vasectomy. Br J Surg 1976;63:477–8.

44. Labrecque M, Pile J, Sokal D, et al. Vasectomy surgical techniques in South and South East Asia. BMC Urol 2005;5:10.

45. Lemack GE, Goldstein M. Presence of sperm in the pre-vasectomy reversal semen analysis: incidence and implications. J Urol 1996;155:167–9.

46. Jaffe TM, Kim ED, Hoekstra TH, et al. Sperm pellet analysis: a technique to detect the presence of sperm in men considered to have azoospermia by routine semen analysis. J Urol 1998;159: 1548–50.

47. Smith JC, Cranston D, O'Brien T, et al. Fatherhood without apparent spermatozoa after vasectomy. Lancet 1994;344:30.

48. Thomson JA, Lincoln PJ, Mortimer P. Paternity by a seemingly infertile vasectomised man. BMJ 1993;307:299–300.

49. Lucon M, Lucon AM, Pasqualoto FF, et al. Paternity after vasectomy with two previous semen analyses without spermatozoa. Sao Paulo Med J 2007;125: 122–3.

50. Labrecque M, Dufresne C, Barone MA, et al. Vasectomy surgical techniques: a systematic review. BMC Med 2004;2:21.

51. Cook LA, Van Vliet H, Lopez LM, et al. Vasectomy occlusion techniques for male sterilization. Cochrane Database Syst Rev 2007;2:CD003991.

52. Kotwal S, Sundaram SK, Rangaiah CS, et al. Does the type of suture material used for ligation of the vas deferens affect vasectomy success? Eur J Contracept Reprod Health Care 2008;13:25–30.

53. Schmidt SS. Vasectomy: principles and comments. J Fam Pract 1991;33:571–3.

54. Reynolds RD. Vas deferens occlusion during no-scalpel vasectomy. J Fam Pract 1994;39:577–82.

55. Goldstein M. Surgical management of male infertility and other scrotal disorders. In: Walsh P, Retik A, Vaughan E, et al, editors. Campbell's urology. 8th edition. Philadelphia: W.B. Saunders Co.; 2002. p. 1532–87.

56. Labrecque M, Nazerali H, Mondor M, et al. Effectiveness and complications associated with 2 vasectomy occlusion techniques. J Urol 2002;168: 2495–8 [discussion: 2498].

57. Mridha SN, Ganguly MM, Jana BR. A study on post-operative vasectomy cases. J Indian Med Assoc 1979;73:209–12.

58. Edwards IS. Follow up after vasectomy. Med J Aust 1973;2:132–5.

59. Mueller-Schmid P, Reimann-Hunziker R, Reimann-Hunziker G. Experiences with sterilization of the male. Praxis 1960;49:352–6.

60. Carlson HE. Vasectomy of election. South Med J 1970;63:766–70.

61. Craft I, Diggory P. Sperm-counts after vasectomy. Lancet 1973;1:995–6.

62. Denniston GC. Vasectomy by electrocautery: outcomes in a series of 2,500 patients. J Fam Pract 1985;21:35–40.

63. Labrecque M, Hoang DQ, Turcot L. Association between the length of the vas deferens excised during vasectomy and the risk of postvasectomy recanalization. Fertil Steril 2003;79:1003–7.

64. Kirby D, Utz WJ, Parks PJ. An implantable ligation device that achieves male sterilization without cutting the vas deferens. Urology 2006;67:807–11.

65. Levine LA, Abern MR, Lux MM. Persistent motile sperm after ligation band vasectomy. J Urol 2006; 176:2146–8.

66. Aradhya KW, Best K, Sokal DC. Recent developments in vasectomy. BMJ 2005;330:296–9.

67. Schmidt SS. Prevention of failure in vasectomy. J Urol 1973;109:296–7.

68. Rhodes DB, Mumford SD, Free MJ. Vasectomy: efficacy of placing the cut vas in different fascial planes. Fertil Steril 1980;33:433–8.

69. Li SQ, Xu B, Hou YH, et al. Relationship between vas occlusion techniques and recanalization. Adv Contracept Deliv Syst 1994;10:153–9.

70. De Los Rios Osorio J, Arenas A, De Los Rios Osorio S. Vasectomy without interposition of fascia is a disaster. Urologia Colombiana 1994;4:14–9.

71. De los Rios Osorio J, Castro Alvarez EA. [Analysis of 5000 vasectomies at a family planning clinic in Medellin-Colombia]. Arch Esp Urol 2003;56:53–60 [in Spanish].

72. Bangstrup L, Pedersen ML. [Sterilization of men. Comparison of 3 different surgical methods]. Ugeskr Laeger 1977;139:1476–8 [in Danish].

73. Shapiro EI, Silber SJ. Open-ended vasectomy, sperm granuloma, and postvasectomy orchialgia. Fertil Steril 1979;32:546–50.

74. Philp T, Guillebaud J, Budd D. Complications of vasectomy: review of 16,000 patients. Br J Urol 1984;56:745–8.

75. Sokal D, Irsula B, Chen-Mok M, et al. A comparison of vas occlusion techniques: cautery more effective than ligation and excision with fascial interposition. BMC Urol 2004;4:12.

76. Moss WM. A sutureless technic for bilateral partial vasectomy. Fertil Steril 1972;23:33–7.

77. Moss WM. Sutureless vasectomy, an improved technique: 1300 cases performed without failure. Fertil Steril 1976;27:1040–5.

78. Moss WM. A comparison of open-end versus closed-end vasectomies: a report on 6220 cases. Contraception 1992;46(6):521–5, 92.

79. Schmidt SS, Free MJ. The bipolar needle for vasectomy. I. Experience with the first 1000 cases. Fertil Steril 1978;29:676–80.

80. Esho JO, Cass AS. Recanalization rate following methods of vasectomy using interposition of fascial sheath of vas deferens. J Urol 1978;120:178–9.

81. Simcock BW. A comparison of three vasectomy techniques in Australia. In: Proceedings of the First National Conference on Surgical Contraception. Sri Lanka: Sri Lanka Association for Voluntary Sterilization; 1978. p. 134–40.

82. Labrecque M, Bedard L, Laperriere L. [Efficacy and complications associated with vasectomies in two clinics in the Quebec region]. Can Fam Physician 1998;44:1860–6 [in French].

83. Schmidt SS, Minckler TM. The vas after vasectomy: comparison of cauterization methods. Urology 1992; 40:468–70.

84. Black T, Francome C. The evolution of the Marie Stopes electrocautery no-scalpel vasectomy procedure. J Fam Plann Reprod Health Care 2002;28: 137–8.

85. Labrecque M, Caron C: Effectiveness of intraluminal thermal cautery alone without cutting the vas: preliminary results. In: Proceedings of the International Conference on Men as Partners in Sexual and Reproductive Health, Mumbai, India, November 28-December 1, 2004.

86. Gupta AS, Kothari LK, Devpura TP. Vas occlusion by tantalum clips and its comparison with conventional vasectomy in man: reliability, reversibility, and complications. Fertil Steril 1977;28:1086–9.

87. Clausen S, Lindenberg S, Nielsen ML, et al. A randomized trial of vas occlusion versus vasectomy for male contraception. Scand J Urol Nephrol 1983; 17:45–6.

88. Whyte J, Cisneros AI, Rubio E, et al. Morphometric study of testis of Wistar rat after open-ended vasectomy. Clin Anat 2002;15:335–9.

89. Errey BB, Edwards IS. Open-ended vasectomy: an assessment. Fertil Steril 1986;45:843–6.

Risks and Complications of Vasectomy

Christopher E. Adams, MD, Moshe Wald, MD*

KEYWORDS
- Vasectomy • Sterilization • Reproductive
- Postoperative complications • Hematoma
- Wound infection • Orchitis

Vasectomy remains an important tool in the armamentarium of contraception. A large historical cohort study revealed that approximately 12% of men aged 12 to 39 have undergone vasectomy.[1] There are approximately 500,000 vasectomies done in the United States yearly, making vasectomy the most common urologic procedure done in this country.[2] Worldwide, 42 to 60 million men use vasectomy as their primary method of contraception.[3] The number of vasectomies performed in the United States and globally, however, pales in comparison to tubal ligation. In 2002, female sterilization done in the United States outnumbered vasectomy by a margin of 3 to 1 (27% versus 9%);[4] this margin also approximately holds true globally.[5]

According to a 2004 study, vasectomy costs seem lower than those associated with tubal ligation in the United States.[4] The same study also found that vasectomy was 30 times less likely to fail and 20 times less likely to have postoperative complications.

Vasectomy is considered a safe and effective way to deliver permanent sterilization. Additionally, 72% of the vasectomies in the United States are performed by urologists. Nevertheless, vasectomy is still a surgical procedure and, as such, has appreciable complications and long-term morbidity. Complications of the procedure include hematoma formation, infection, failed sterilization, sperm granuloma, short-term incisional pain, and chronic pain syndromes. Another possible consequence of vasectomy is the development of antisperm antibodies. This article discusses in detail the prevalence of these risks,

how variations in surgical technique affect complications, and how current pathophysiology explains some of the complications.

HEMATOMA FORMATION

The most common immediate complication of vasectomy is hematoma formation. Scrotal hematoma is aesthetically displeasing and painful during the postoperative course. The incidence of scrotal hematoma after vasectomy is low. The accepted overall incidence for hematoma formation is 2% (range, 0.09%–29%).[6] According to a national survey of vasectomy providers, the incidence of scrotal hematoma is directly related to the number of vasectomies completed by a physician annually and was reported to be 4.6% for physicians performing 1 to 10 vasectomies annually, 2.4% for those performing 11 to 50 annually, and 1.6% for those performing more than 50 annually. Physician experience also correlates with hospitalization with incidences of 0.8%, 0.3%, and 0.2%, respectively.[3,6]

One of the factors that influences hematoma occurrence involves the chosen surgical technique, more specifically, no-scalpel vasectomy versus traditional incisional vasectomy. The no-scalpel vasectomy technique has been reported associated with a lower incidence of bleeding and hematoma formation compared with the standard incisional technique. Two randomized controlled studies have demonstrated this advantage. A pivotal study done by Sokal and colleagues[7] showed an 85% reduction in the frequency of hematoma formation (1.8% versus

Department of Urology, University of Iowa, 200 Hawkins Drive, 3 RCP, Iowa City, IA 52242-1089, USA
* Corresponding author.
E-mail address: moshe-wald@uiowa.edu (M. Wald).

Urol Clin N Am 36 (2009) 331–336
doi:10.1016/j.ucl.2009.05.009

12%). In this study, two of the three hospitalizations required after vasectomy were related to hematoma formation. Christensen and colleagues[8] had a much smaller patient population but showed a reduction of hematoma formation with no-scalpel (9.5%) versus standard incision (15.9%).[9] Sokal and colleagues[7] also showed a decrease in perioperative bleeding with no-scalpel (2.1%) versus standard incision (4.29%). As the scrotum is expandable and has poor tamponading characteristics, strict hemostasis at the end of the procedure, regardless of technique, is essential to prevent hematoma. Postoperative care, including elevation of the scrotum and compressive dressings, also plays an important role in reducing postoperative bleeding. Some studies recommend suturing the scrotum to the abdominal wall or use of scrotal hitches to prevent subcutaneous tracking of blood, but this is not common practice.[10,11]

VASECTOMY FAILURE

The failure to achieve or maintain sterilization is one of the most devastating risks of vasectomy. In general, vasectomy failure is defined by the presence of sperm in the ejaculate after the procedure, but the actual definitions vary in terms of sperm numbersand time after vasectomy. For example, although some investigators define vasectomy failure as more than 10 million sperm/L at 12 weeks or later, others define it as more than 5 million motile sperm/mL at 14 weeks or later or more than 100 000 sperm/mL with any motility at 26 weeks or later.[12] It is recommended, however, that if any motile sperm are found in the ejaculate 3 months after vasectomy, the procedure should be repeated.[2] Unwanted pregnancy can place major strains on couples and be a source of litigation against the practicing physician. Pregnancy rates associated with failure are reported to range from 0% to 2%.[13] There is no absolute standard of care for the confirmation of postvasectomy sterility. Follow-up semen analysis is recommended 2 to 3 months after vasectomy, with the goal of obtaining at least one and preferably two absolutely azoospermic specimens 4 to 6 weeks apart.[2] Vasectomy failure can be a result of a surgical error, such as disrupting or occluding a structure other than the vas deferens, incomplete disruption of the vas, failure to recognize duplications of the vas deferens, or repeating a vasectomy on the same vas.[14] Practicing unprotected sexual intercourse too soon after a vasectomy also represents a potential cause of failed sterilization.

When appropriate disruption of both vasa deferentia is accomplished and sufficient time before resuming unprotected sexual intercourse is allowed, however, recanalization of the vas deferens may be the cause of vasectomy failure. Knowledge of the recanalization process is based on histopathologic studies. Tissue samples obtained from men undergoing vasectomy reversal have shown epithelialized microtubules on both abdominal and testicular vasal ends; sperm has been observed within the microtubules themselves or extravasating from them.[15,16] A novel experiment by Stahl and coworkers[17] showed statistically significant up-regulation of selected growth factors at vasectomy sites, although a direct mechanism of microrecanalization could not be elicited. Further studies are needed to delineate the exact mechanism of postvasectomy microrecanalization.

The most heavily debated source of failed sterilization stems from the surgical technique used for vasectomy. Disruption of the vas represents the most important step to achieve permanent sterilization. Many techniques have been described in the literature with associated failure rates. Worldwide, the most commonly used technique is simple suture ligation with excision.[12] Although vasectomy traditionally has been believed to have overall failure rates of 1% to 3% or lower, recent studies indicate higher failure rates for the ligation and excision technique.[12] A large, multinational, randomized trial showed that ligation and excision plus fascial interposition (**Fig. 1**) is significantly more effective than ligation and excision alone.[18] Addition of fascial interposition to suture ligation with vasal excision lowered the failure rate (defined in that study as more than 5 million motile sperm/mL at 14 weeks or later or more than 100 000 sperm/mL with any motility at 26 weeks or later) from 12.7% to 5.9%.[12] A common explanation for this failure rate involves tip necrosis and sloughing secondary to ligation; this is turn leads to recanalization of the cut vas segments.[19]

Failure rates seem to decrease dramatically with use of fascial interposition and use of electrocautery. A retrospective Canadian study reported an 8.7% failure rate with clip ligation and excision

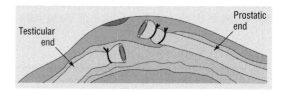

Fig. 1. Fascial interposition. (*From* Aradhya KW, Best K, Sokal DC. Recent developments in vasectomy. BMJ 2005;330(7486):296; with permission.)

without fascial interposition; however, the same study found that cautery with fascial interposition had approximately a 0.3% failure rate.[20] Dassow and Bennett compiled a variety of vasectomy techniques with corresponding failure rates based on comparative literature review (**Table 1**).

POSTVASECTOMY PAIN

Short-term pain is to be expected after vasectomy. Approximately 30% of patients report some type of pain even 2 to 3 weeks after surgery.[21] Long-term pain requiring more aggressive medical or surgical intervention, however, is expected in 1 out 1000 men who undergo a vasectomy.[2] Congestive epididymitis and chronic orchalgia are uncommon postvasectomy complications. They comprise a chronic pain syndrome often recognized as postvasectomy pain syndrome (PVPS).[22] Congestive epididymitis is a rare event, reported in only 0.4% to 6.1% of vasectomies.[23,24] Congestive epididymitis usually presents as testicular or scrotal tenderness on the affected side; pain usually lasts weeks to months with only rare cases lasting greater than 1 year.[3] Congestive epididymitis is believed the result of elevated pressures in closed-ended vasectomy. Thus, mechanical pressure, not inflammation, is the cause of the pain. Histologic findings in patients who have scrotal pain show epididymal engorgement, complex cystic disease, and chronic changes of epididymitis. Cultures from excised epididymis support the notion that pain is not caused by infectious etiologies.[1,25,26] A study comparing open-ended versus closed-ended vasectomy showed a higher rate of congestive epididymitis for closed-ended vasectomy (6% versus 2%; relative risk 3.0 [95% CI, 1.2–7.5]).[27] Additionally, one study reported variations among direct closed-ended techniques. Ligation of both

testicular and abdominal ends resulted in an incidence of 5.6% (288 procedures), whereas bipolar (1000 cases) and monopolar (1600) cautery resulted in an incidence of 3.8% and 2.8%, respectively.[28]

Conservative measures should be first-line therapy for management of PVPS. Scrotal elevation, scrotal support, hot and cold compressions, activity restrictions (strenuous and sexual), and oral analgesics play an important role in the initial management of this type of scrotal pain. Empirically prescribed antibiotic therapy likely has limited effect, as suggested by reported histopathologic findings that are not consistent with infection.[26] If conservative measures fail, more aggressive medical therapies may be helpful. Spermatic cord blocks or use of local steroid injections can provide symptomatic relief.[2] Tricyclic antidepressants have had limited success in some case reports. Transrectal injections of bupivacaine and methylprednisolone into the pelvic plexus have been used as a treatment option.[29]

Several surgical options are available for the management of chronic testicular pain when conservative and medical measures are unsuccessful. Epididymectomy, vasectomy reversal, denervation of the spermatic cord, and orchiectomy all have been studied as possible treatments of chronic orchalgia. One series reported up to 50% cure rate with surgical removal of the epididymis, vas deferens, and corresponding scar tissues.[30] Nangia and colleagues[31] reported 69% cure rate for patients undergoing vasectomy reversal for postvasectomy pain; the obvious drawback to this treatment is the loss of desired sterility. Both studies emphasized the importance of appropriate patient selection for obtaining improved results. Levine and Matkov reported good pain-free outcomes after denervation of the spermatic cord.[32] Their surgical technique

Table 1	
Failure rates of vasectomy by surgical technique[a]	
Surgical Technique	**Reported Failure Rates**
Cautery and excision	≤4.8%
Cautery and fascial interpostion	≤1.2%
Ligation and fascial interposition	≤16.7
Intraluminal cautery	<1%
Ligation and excision	1.5%–29%
Cautery (open testicular end) and fascial interposition	0.02–2.4%

[a] Failure defined as presence of sperm.
Data from Dassow P, Bennett JM. Vasectomy: an update. Am Fam Physician 2006;74(12):2069–74.

included microsurgical division of the ilioinguinal nerve and its branches, vas deferens division to ensure sympathetic denervation, and transection of all tissues except one artery (cremasteric, deferential, or testicular) and one lymphatic vessel. The patients selected for this procedure were those who had some form of relief from spermatic cord block and normal physical examination. Of a cohort of 27 patients, 76% reported complete resolution of symptoms, with partial relief in another 9%. This group recently studied the long-term outcomes of this procedure and reported durable pain relief in 71% of testicular units, partial relief in 17%, and unchanged pain in 12%, with no patients having worse pain.[33] Finally, orchiectomy has been reported as a last resort for patients who have refractory testicular pain when conservative measures are unsuccessful. In a study of patients who had chronic orchalgia of varying etiologies, Davis and colleagues[34] reported better results with inguinal versus scrotal orchiectomy (73% versus 55%) for intractable testicular pain.

SPERM GRANULOMA

Sperm granulomas are inflammatory reactions that occur in response to extravasated sperm. They have been identified in 15% to 40% of specimens obtained during vasectomy reversals.[35] A majority of the sperm granulomas remain asymptomatic. A small subset (2%–3%) of vasectomy patients has pain that can be attributed to sperm granuloma, usually occurring 2 to 3 weeks postoperatively.[3] Vasitis nodosa is another complication of vasectomy that is closely related to sperm granulomas. This condition is characterized by a localized proliferation of ductal structures after injury to the vas deferens and typically is detected as an incidental histologic finding at the time of a vasectomy reversal.[3]

INFECTION

Infection after vasectomy is a recognized complication affecting approximately 3.5% of patients. Much variation exists, especially between no-scalpel versus traditional incisional technique. One randomized controlled study reported a 0.2% infection rate with no-scalpel technique versus 1.5% for standard incisional vasectomy.[7] Another study showed infection rates of no-scalpel versus incisional vasectomy techniques as 7.1% and 11.4%, respectively.[8] Most infections are limited and treated with a simple course of antibiotics. Scrotal cleansing is used at the surgeon's discretion, and the scrotum should be shaved at the time of surgery. More systemic infections stemming from vasectomy are rare. There are case reports of Fournier's gangrene after vasectomy[36] and infective endocarditis.[37]

IMMUNOLOGIC EFFECTS OF VASECTOMY

Another common consequence of vasectomy is the development of antisperm antibodies. Vasectomy may cause sperm antigens to be exposed to the immune system, resulting in an antisperm autoantibody response.[38,39] In a recent study, 240 of 272 (88%) men who had a history of prior vasectomy were found to possess serum antisperm antibodies.[40] Many studies have addressed the relationship between immune-complex diseases and antisperm autoantibodies. Massey and colleagues[1] followed 10,590 men with paired controls (median 7.9-year follow-up) and found no increase in immune-complex diseases, such as systemic lupus erythematous, scleroderma, or rheumatoid arthritis, and found the only significant increase in disease incidence was epididymitis/orchitis. Another study of 23,988 vasectomized men and 146,000 matched controls compared immune-complex disease incidence in vasectomized men with matched controls over approximately 12 years of follow-up.[41] This study concluded that there was no long-term elevation in risk for asthma, inflammatory bowel disease, ankylosing spondylitis, and certain other immune-related diseases after vasectomy. The only disease associated with elevated risk, again, was epididymitis/orchitis.[41] Although these aforementioned studies do not suggest that the sequelae of antisperm antibodies is associated with an increased risk for immune-related diseases, these antibodies may impair sperm function in men who become interested in resuming their fertility through a vasectomy reversal.[39]

SUMMARY

Urologists will remain an important provider of sterilization for undesired fertility. Vasectomy is a safe and effective procedure for permanent contraception and is an important component of urologic practice. Compared with its gynecologic counterpart, vasectomy is 30 times less likely to fail and 20 times less likely to have postoperative complications. Complications from vasectomy, fortunately, are rare, and mostly minor in nature. Immediate risks include infection, hematoma, and pain. Although bothersome, these complications seldom lead to hospitalization or more aggressive medical management. Case reports exist concerning Fournier's gangrene and endocarditis after vasectomy but should not warrant much counsel between provider and patient due to the reported rarity of these conditions. Although most hospitalizations after vasectomy are for hematoma management, a majority of hematomas can be treated conservatively and prevented with strict surgical hemostasis. Chronic pain syndromes (PVPS) have effective medical treatments and surgical forms of relief have good results in select patients; fortunately, PVPS is infrequent. Surgical technique is surgeon dependent and to be respected; however, certain surgical techniques, such as fascial interposition, seem to decrease rates of vasectomy failure. Despite myriad vasectomy techniques, overall failure rates are far less than those seen with tubal ligation. Antisperm antibodies are found in more than 60% of vasectomized men, but current available data suggest that these men do not seem at increased risk for immune-complex diseases.

REFERENCES

1. Massey FJ, Bernstein GS, O'Fallon WM, et al. Vasectomy and health. Results from a large cohort study. JAMA 1984;252(8):1023–9.

2. Sandlow JI, Winfield HN, Goldstein M. Surgery of the scrotum and seminal vesicles. In: Wein AJ, Kavoussi LR, Novick AC, et al, editors. Campbell-Walsh urology. 9th edition. Philadelphia: Saunders; 2007. p. 1098–127, chapter 34.

3. Schwingl PJ, Guess HA. Safety and effectiveness of vasectomy. Fertil Steril 2000;73(5):923–36.

4. Mosher WD, Martinez GM, Chandra A, et al. Use of contraception and use of family planning services in the United States: 1982–2002. Adv Data 2004;Dec (350):1–36.

5. Hendrix NW, Chauhan SP, Morrison JC. Sterilization and its consequences. Obstet Gynecol Surv 1999; 54(12):766–77.

6. Kendrick JS, Gonzales B, Huber DH, et al. Complications of vasectomies in the United States. J Fam Pract 1987;25(3):245–8.

7. Sokal D, McMullen S, Gates D, et al. A comparative study of the no scalpel and standard incision approaches to vasectomy in 5 countries. The Male Sterilization Investigator Team. J Urol 1999;162(5): 1621–5.

8. Christensen P, al-Aqidi OA, Jensen FS, et al. Vasectomy. A prospective, randomized trial of vasectomy with bilateral incision versus the Li vasectomy. Ugeskr Laeger 2002;164(18):2390–4.

9. Cook LA, Pun A, van Vliet H, et al. Scalpel versus no-scalpel incision for vasectomy. Cochrane Database Syst Rev 2007;(2):CD004112.

10. Griffin JH, Canning JR. The scrotal hitch for hemostasis and edema prevention in scrotal surgery. Urology 1996;47(6):918–9.

11. Oesterling JE. Scrotal surgery: a reliable method for the prevention of postoperative hematoma and edema. J Urol 1990;143(6):1201–2.

12. Aradhya KW, Best K, Sokal DC. Recent developments in vasectomy. BMJ 2005;330(7486):296–9.

13. Dassow P, Bennett JM. Vasectomy: an update. Am Fam Physician 2006;74(12):2069–74.

14. Labrecque M, Hays M, Chen-Mok M, et al. Frequency and patterns of early recanalization after vasectomy. BMC Urol 2006;6:25.

15. Freund MJ, Weidmann JE, Goldstein M, et al. Micro-recanalization after vasectomy in man. J Androl 1989;10(2):120–32.

16. Cruickshank B, Eidus L, Barkin M. Regeneration of vas deferens after vasectomy. Urology 1987;30(2): 137–42.

17. Stahl BC, Ratliff TL, De Young BR, et al. Involvement of growth factors in the process of post-vasectomy micro-recanalization. J Urol 2008;179(1):376–80.

18. Sokal D, Irsula B, Hays M, et al. Investigator Study Group. Vasectomy by ligation and excision, with or without fascial interposition: a randomized controlled trial. BMC Med 2004;2:6.

19. Schmidt SS. Techniques and complications of elective vasectomy. The role of spermatic granuloma in spontaneous recanalization. Fertil Steril 1966;17(4):467–82.

20. Labrecque M, Nazerali H, Mondor M, et al. Effectiveness and complications associated with 2 vasectomy occlusion techniques. J Urol 2002;168(6):2495–8.

21. Tandon S, Sabanegh E Jr. Chronic pain after vasectomy: a diagnostic and treatment dilemma. BJU Int 2008;102(2):166–9.

22. Christiansen CG, Sandlow JI. Testicular pain following vasectomy: a review of postvasectomy pain syndrome. J Androl 2003;24(3):293–8.

23. Raspa RF. Complications of vasectomy. Am Fam Physician 1993;48(7):1264–8.

24. Schmidt SS. Vasectomy by section, luminal fulguration and fascial interposition: results from 6248 cases. Br J Urol 1995;76(3):373–5.

25. West AF, Leung HY, Powell PH. Epididymectomy is an effective treatment for scrotal pain after vasectomy. BJU Int 2000;85(9):1097–9.

26. Selikowitz SM, Schned AR. A late post-vasectomy syndrome. J Urol 1985;134(3):494–7.

27. Moss WM. A comparison of open-end versus closed-end vasectomies: a report on 6220 cases. Contraception 1992;46(6):521–5.

28. Schmidt SS, Free MJ. The bipolar needle for vasectomy. I. Experience with the first 1000 cases. Fertil Steril 1978;29(6):676–80.

29. Yamamoto M, Hibi H, Katsuno S, et al. Management of chronic orchialgia of unknown etiology. Int J Urol 1995;2(1):47–9.

30. Chen TF, Ball RY. Epididymectomy for post-vasectomy pain: histological review. Br J Urol 1991; 68(4):407–13.

31. Nangia AK, Myles JL, Thomas AJ Jr. Vasectomy reversal for the post-vasectomy pain syndrome: a clinical and histological evaluation. J Urol 2000; 164(6):1939–42.

32. Levine LA, Matkov TG. Microsurgical denervation of the spermatic cord as primary surgical treatment of chronic orchialgia. J Urol 2001;165(6 Pt 1): 1927–9.

33. Strom KH, Levine LA. Microsurgical denervation of the spermatic cord for chronic orchialgia: long-term results from a single center. J Urol 2008; 180(3):949–53.

34. Davis BE, Noble MJ, Weigel JW, et al. Analysis and management of chronic testicular pain. J Urol 1990; 143(5):936–9.

35. Balogh K, Argényi ZB. Vasitis nodosa and spermatic granuloma of the skin: an histologic study of a rare complication of vasectomy. J Cutan Pathol 1985; 12(6):528–33.

36. Viddeleer AC, Lycklama Á, Nijeholt GA. Lethal Fournier's gangrene following vasectomy. J Urol 1992; 147(6):1613–4.

37. Kessler RB, Kimbrough RC 3rd, Jones SR. Infective endocarditis caused by Staphylococcus hominis after vasectomy. Clin Infect Dis 1998;27(1):216–7.

38. Lepow IH, Crozier R, editors. Vasectomy: immunologic and pathophysiologic effects in animals and man. London: Academic Press; 1979. p. 267–84.

39. Sotolongo JR Jr. Immunologic effects of vasectomy. J Urol 1982;127(6):1063–6.

40. Lee R, Goldstein M, Ullery BW, et al. Value of serum antisperm antibodies in diagnosing obstructive azoospermia. J Urol 2009;181(1):264–9.

41. Goldacre MJ, Wotton CJ, Seagroatt V, et al. Immune-related disease before and after vasectomy: an epidemiological database study. Humanit Rep 2007;22(5):1273–8.

Putative Health Risks Associated with Vasectomy

Tobias S. Köhler, MD, MPH[a], Anees A. Fazili, MD[b],
Robert E. Brannigan, MD[b],*

KEYWORDS
- Vasectomy • Vasectomy complications • Prostate cancer
- Primary progressive aphasia • Health risks

Historically, many authors have reported concerns regarding the safety of vasectomy. Prior studies have linked vasectomy with a number of health risks, including the development of cardiovascular disease, testicular cancer, prostate cancer, psychologic distress, and a variety of immune complex–mediated disease processes.[1–8] In the case of each of these reported risks, subsequent research has generally failed to show convincing association between vasectomy and the conditions in question. This subsequent research has been characterized by more adequately powered, appropriately designed studies better able to control for potential bias and confounding variables. This article thoughtfully reviews the literature regarding the health concerns purportedly associated with vasectomy. Also discussed is the recently reported association between vasectomy and primary progressive aphasia (PPA), which to date has not been critically assessed in the medical literature.

CARDIOVASCULAR DISEASE

The initial reports of an association between vasectomy and cardiovascular disease were made in studies conducted by Clarkson and Alexander.[9,10] These authors observed that two different species of vasectomized monkeys (*Macaca fascicularis* and *Macaca mulatta*) had more extensive atherosclerosis compared with age-matched controls, and they speculated that this difference was the result of circulating anti-sperm antibody immune complexes that exacerbated atherosclerosis. Follow-up studies, including one by the original authors, Clarkson and Alexander, failed to substantiate the initial reported association between vasectomy and atherosclerosis.[11,12] Campbell and colleagues[13] investigated the possible link between vasectomy and cardiovascular disease in humans by assessing the distensibility of posterior tibial arteries using Doppler ultrasonographic techniques. The authors reported that men who had undergone prior vasectomy had reduced posterior tibial artery distensibility compared with controls, and they concluded that vasectomized men may be at risk for accelerated development of peripheral arterial disease.

Numerous subsequent studies in humans have dispelled an association between vasectomy and cardiovascular disease.[14–22] These studies collectively assessed a large array of specific cardiovascular parameters, including blood pressure, angiographically determined atherosclerosis, coronary heart disease, myocardial infarction, and death from cardiovascular disease. In sum, these studies concluded that patients who had undergone vasectomy were not at increased cardiovascular risk compared with controls. Even in patients who are 20 or more years postvasectomy, no increase in atherosclerosis or coronary heart disease has been observed.[23] Finally, Kisker and colleagues[24] assessed parameters that could

[a] Division of Urology, Southern Illinois University, 747 North Rutledge, No. 9649, Springfield, IL 62702, USA
[b] Department of Urology, Northwestern University, Feinberg School of Medicine, 303 East Chicago Avenue, Tarry 16-703, Chicago, IL 60611, USA
* Corresponding author.
E-mail address: r-brannigan@northwestern.edu (R.E. Brannigan).

Urol Clin N Am 36 (2009) 337–345
doi:10.1016/j.ucl.2009.05.004
0094-0143/09/$ – see front matter © 2009 Elsevier Inc. All rights reserved.

predispose patients to thrombotic events, including blood coagulation factors, thrombin monomer, and circulating platelet aggregate ratios. The authors found no differences in these markers of thrombotic disease when comparing men who had undergone vasectomy with controls.

OTHER POSTULATED CIRCULATING IMMUNE COMPLEX DISORDERS

Two small studies in rabbits and macaques reported an association between vasectomy and glomerulonephritis, and the authors postulated that circulating immune complex deposition was the mediating factor.[7,25] Several subsequent investigations failed to show any changes in renal function suggestive of glomerulonephritis or any increased prevalence of glomerulonephritis among vasectomized men when compared with nonvasectomized men.[26–28] Repeated studies have also failed to substantiate the initial concerns of circulating immune complex formation induced by postvasectomy antisperm antibodies, because circulating immune complexes were not found to be persistently elevated in men who underwent vasectomy when compared with controls.[29,30] A recent study with a mean follow-up of 13 years similarly demonstrated that men who underwent vasectomy had no long-term increased risk for several other immune system–related diseases, such as ankylosing spondylitis, asthma, diabetes, inflammatory bowel disease, multiple sclerosis, myasthenia gravis, rheumatoid arthritis, or thyrotoxicosis.[31] The significance of antisperm antibodies in vasectomized men is still unclear, but they have not been definitively associated with any pathologic processes aside from the desired result of male sterility.[32,33]

TESTICULAR CANCER

Observations regarding a possible association between vasectomy and testicular cancer were first reported in a 1988 case-control study by Strader and colleagues[5] conducted in western Washington state. On closer analysis, however, the association between vasectomy and testicular cancer in this study was noted to be present only in Catholic men and was speculated to be caused by bias in underreporting a history of vasectomy by Catholic controls. The possibility of an association between vasectomy and testicular cancer reemerged when Thornhill and colleagues,[34] from Ireland and Cale and colleagues[35] from Scotland reported that the risk of testicular cancer may be elevated after vasectomy. Both studies were small, with the first reporting on three patients

and the second reporting on eight patients diagnosed with testicular cancer shortly after vasectomy. The authors of each of these studies suggested that vasectomy may accelerate the growth of an existing tumor, whereas Jorgensen and colleagues[36] in a subsequent manuscript hypothesized that vasectomy may facilitate the development of testicular cancer from previously present carcinoma in situ, a preinvasive lesion. In 1994, Moller and colleagues[37] attempted to clarify the relationship between vasectomy and testicular cancer using computerized linkage of four population-based registers in Denmark. The authors compared cancer rates among the cohort of men who had undergone vasectomy with the whole Danish population. The authors found no increase in testicular cancer in the cohort of 73,917 vasectomized men. They concluded that vasectomy is neither likely to induce testicular tumorigenesis, nor to accelerate the growth and diagnosis of noninvasive precursor lesions or clinically unrecognized tumors. In 1994, the United Kingdom Testicular Cancer Study Group published a population-based case-control study on the etiology of testicular cancer involving 794 men from nine health regions in England and Wales.[38] The authors found no association between vasectomy and testicular cancer. These final two studies are the largest to date, and both effectively dispel the notion that vasectomy is associated with testicular cancer.

PROSTATE CANCER

In 1990, two separate case-control studies by Rosenberg and colleagues[2] and Mettlin and colleagues[1] generated significant debate by reporting an association between vasectomy and prostate cancer. These two studies supported the finding of an association between vasectomy and prostate cancer that was initially reported by Honda and colleagues[39] in 1988. Critics were quick to note, however, that the control group in the study by Rosenberg and colleagues[2] had a vasectomy rate far below the general population. They contended that the apparent bias in the control group exaggerated potential differences between cases and controls.[40] A follow-up study by the original authors with better accounting for this bias revealed no association between vasectomy and prostate cancer.[41] Despite this follow-up report, numerous subsequent studies by other groups also suggested an association between vasectomy and prostate cancer (**Table 1**). These studies have been criticized as suffering from some degree of detection bias or surveillance bias, because men who have undergone vasectomy typically have access to a urologist and are more likely to be screened for prostate cancer.[42–44] Other studies associating vasectomy and prostate cancer have been plagued by similar problems of selection bias stemming from an overall differential access to health care between cases and controls. This is a reflection of the fact that vasectomies in the United States are generally performed on men of higher socioeconomic backgrounds who have good access to health care and frequently use health care resources.[45,46]

The issue of possible confounding has also been noted in studies reporting links between vasectomy and prostate cancer. This was illustrated in 1993 when two separate cohort studies from Giovannucci and colleagues[3,4] in the *Journal of the American Medical Association* demonstrated an association between vasectomy and prostate cancer. According to these studies, the age-adjusted relative risk for prostate cancer among men with vasectomies was 1.66 (95% confidence interval [CI], 1.25–2.21) and 1.56 (95% CI, 1.03–2.37). In an editorial within the same issue of the *Journal of the American Medical Association*, Howards and Peterson[47] wrote that the most likely noncausal explanation for Giovannucci and colleagues[3,4] findings was unmeasured confounding, based on the fact that the specific etiology of prostate cancer remains unknown. In 1996, Sandlow and Kreder[48] surveyed 1500 urologists regarding the impact of reports of an association between vasectomy and prostate cancer on urologists' practice patterns. Although 90% of the 759 respondents noted that these reports had little or no effect on their practice of vasectomy, 27% acknowledged that they screened vasectomized men earlier from prostate cancer. Additionally, 20% responded that they are reluctant to recommend a vasectomy to a man with a strong family history of prostate cancer. The authors concluded that over one fourth of the urologists who screen for prostate cancer altered their screening patterns, despite responding that the studies had not affected their practice patterns.

In the years that followed, multiple studies failed to find an association between vasectomy and prostate cancer (see **Table 1**). Of these, perhaps the most notable was a large population-based, case-control study from New Zealand that was published in 1992 and compared 923 prostate cancer patients with 1224 matched controls. Although a case-control design, this study benefited from its large population sample. New Zealand has the highest vasectomy prevalence in the world, and statutory identification of cancer into a national registry, providing the framework to avoid many potential sources of confounding.

This study found no significantly increased risk of prostate cancer in men with prior vasectomies (RR of 0.92; 95% CI, 0.75–1.14), even after adjusting for patient age, age at vasectomy, time since vasectomy, age of prostate cancer diagnosis, family history of prostate cancer, and stage of cancer.[49] A case-control study specifically designed to address the issue of risk of prostate cancer in specific subgroups was published in 2002.[50] This study assessed 1001 men and revealed no association between prostate cancer and age at vasectomy, years elapsed since vasectomy, family history of prostate cancer, or race. This publication supported the assertion that vasectomy does not lead to an increased risk of prostate cancer, even in men with longer follow-up and in populations at increased risk for this disease, such as African American men or men with a family history of prostate cancer.

MORTALITY

Giovannucci and coworkers'[22] 1992 *New England Journal of Medicine* manuscript reported on a retrospective cohort analysis of husbands from the Nurses' Health Study. The authors compared 14,607 men who had undergone vasectomy as of 1976 with 14,607 men who had not undergone vasectomy. The authors found that vasectomy was neither associated with an increase in overall mortality nor mortality from cardiovascular disease. Although they reported no overall increase in mortality from cancer after vasectomy, they did observe an increased risk for mortality from cancer in men 20 years or more after vasectomy. This finding helped prompt the subsequent closer look at vasectomy and prostate cancer, as discussed previously.

TESTICULAR ANATOMY AND PHYSIOLOGY

Several authors have reported changes in testicular anatomy and physiology after vasectomy. Jarow and colleagues[51] compared testicular morphometry and antisperm antibody status from 19 vasectomized men with 21 fertile control subjects. Vasectomized men were found to have significant increases in seminiferous tubule wall thickness and focal interstitial fibrosis compared with controls. Serum antisperm antibody activity was observed in 74% of the vasectomized men and none of the controls, but no association was found between histologic changes and antibody status. The authors concluded that some other pathophysiologic process besides antisperm antibodies must be responsible for the observed testicular histology changes. Raleigh and

Table 1
Studies evaluating the association between vasectomy and prostate cancer

Author (y)	Study Design	Study Size	Number of Vasectomized Men with Prostate Cancer	Study Conclusions: RR (95% CI)
Honda et al (1988)	Population-based case-control	216 matched case-control pairs	58	RR 1.4 (0.9–2.3) RR 2.2 (1.0–4.8), 20–29 y postvasectomy RR 4.4 (0.9–2.1), ≥30 y postvasectomy
Mettlin et al (1990)	Hospital-based case-control	614 cases, 2588 controls	27	RR 1.7 (1.1–2.6) Age-adj. RR 2.2 (1.0–4.6), 13–18 y postvasectomy
Rosenberg et al (1990)	Hospital-based case-control	220 cases, 960 cancer controls, 571 noncancer controls	22	Age-adj. RR 5.3 (2.7–10) versus noncancer controls Age-adj. RR 3.5 (2.1–6.0) versus cancer controls
Sidney et al (1991)	Retrospective cohort study	5119 vasectomized men; 15,357 controls	68	RR 1.0 (0.7–1.6)
Nienhuis et al (1992)	Retrospective cohort study	13,246 vasectomized men; 22,196 controls	1	RR 0.44 (0.1–4.0)
Giovannucci et al (1993)	Retrospective cohort (husbands of women in Nurses Health Study)	14,607 vasectomized men; 14,607 age-matched controls	54	Age-adj. RR 1.56 (1.03–2.37) RR 1.89 (1.14–3.14), ≥20 y postvasectomy
Giovannucci et al (1993)	Prospective cohort (men from Health Professionals Follow-up Study)	10,055 men with vasectomy; 37,800 controls	59	Age-adj RR 1.66 (1.25–2.21) Age-adj RR 1.56 (1.15–2.11), after excluding stage A1 cases RR 1.85 (1.26–2.72), ≥22 y postvasectomy
Hayes et al (1993)	Population-based case-control	Blacks: 471 cases, 589 controls Whites: 494 cases, 703 controls	Blacks: 7 Whites: 49	All: RR 1.2 (0.8–1.7) Blacks: RR 1.6 (0.5–4.8) Whites: RR 1.1 (0.8–1.7) RR 1.5 (0.8–2.7), ≥20 y postvasectomy (all) RR 1.7 (0.9–3.3), whites ≥20 y postvasectomy RR 2.0 (1.0–4.0), <35 y age at vasectomy (all) RR 2.2 (1.0–4.4), whites <35 y age at vasectomy
Rosenberg et al (1994)	Hospital-based case-control	355 cases, 2048 control	18	RR 1.2 (0.6–2.7) RR 1.4 (0.5–4.2), ≥15 y postvasectomy

Study	Study type	Cases/controls	n	RR (95% CI)
Moller et al (1994)	Registry-based cohort	73,917 vasectomized men; Danish male population (control)	165	RR 0.98 (0.84–1.14)
John et al (1995)	Population-based case-control	1642 cases, 1636 controls	172	All: RR 1.1 (0.83–1.3) Whites: RR 0.94 (0.69–1.3) Blacks: RR 1.0 (0.59–1.8) Chinese-Americans: RR 0.96 (0.42–2.2) Japanese-Americans: RR 1.8 (0.97–3.4)
Zhu et al (1996)	HMO-based case-control	175 cases, 258 controls	61	RR 0.86 (0.57–1.32) RR 0.84 (0.51–1.38), $\geq$20 y postvasectomy
Platz et al (1997)	Hospital-based case-control (hospitals covered by Bombay Cancer Registry)	175 cases, 978 cancer controls	17	Age-adj RR 1.31 (0.74–2.33) RR 1.56 (0.79–3.08), $\geq$20 y postvasectomy RR 2.10 (1.02–4.31), >40 y at time of vasectomy
Stanford et al (1999)	Population-based case-control (Seattle SEER database)	753 cases, 703 controls	297	RR 1.10 (0.9–1.4)
Cox et al (2002)	Population-based case-control (New Zealand Cancer Registry)	923 cases, 1224 controls	216	RR 0.92 (0.75–1.14) RR 0.92 (0.68–1.23), $\geq$25 y postvasectomy RR 0.94 (0.75–1.17), $\geq$T2 stage RR 0.95 (0.64–1.40), + FHx prostate cancer
Holt et al (2008)	Population-based case-control	1001 cases, 942 matched controls	362	RR 1.0 (0.8–1.2) RR 1.1 (0.7–1.7), 20–24 y postvasectomy RR 0.9 (0.6–1.2), 30–34 y postvasectomy RR 0.7 (0.5–1.1), $\geq$35 y postvasectomy

colleagues[52] compared testicular biopsies from 34 men undergoing vasectomy reversal with biopsies from 10 normal men taken at the time of vasectomy. Vasectomized men were observed to have a significant reduction in germ cells in the later stages of spermatogenesis (pachytene spermatocytes and spermatids) and increases in testicular fibrosis. These changes were each more pronounced with increasing obstructive interval, and no association between spermatogenic damage and antisperm antibody status was found. In 2007, O'Neill and colleagues[53] reported that sperm yields from testicular biopsies on vasectomized men (>5 years postvasectomy) compared with fertile men (biopsied at the time of vasectomy) were markedly reduced. The authors found increased germ cell apoptosis and increased sperm DNA fragmentation in the vasectomized men compared with fertile controls. In 2004, Nicopoullos and colleagues[54] evaluated 37 men with a prior history of vasectomy who underwent surgical sperm retrieval for use in in vitro fertilization and intracytoplasmic sperm injection. The outcomes they assessed were fertilization rate, implantation rate, clinical pregnancy rate, and live-birth rate per embryo transfer. The authors observed no effect of time since vasectomy on any outcome. They concluded that maternal age, not interval of time since vasectomy, was the principal determinant of in vitro fertilization and intracytoplasmic sperm injection success.

PSYCHOLOGIC DISTRESS

Numerous studies have assessed the association between vasectomy and subsequent development of postoperative psychologic distress. Potential psychologic sequelae observed in men after vasectomy are fairly broad in scope, and include anxiety, depression, and regret over having the procedure. In a 1990 review, Thonneau and D'Isle[55] concluded that 90% of men are satisfied with having had a vasectomy. Nonetheless, concerns over loss of masculinity after vasectomy and desire to have children in the future do result in psychologic distress in some patients.[56–58] In her 1996 review, Rogstad[57] observed that most studies found that adverse psychologic events were least common in men who made the decision to pursue vasectomy jointly with their spouses. She also reported that possible predictors of psychosexual problems postvasectomy include pre-existing emotional instability, excessive concerns regarding masculinity, confusion of vasectomy with castration, and postoperative complaints. She concluded that major predictors of poststerilization regret are preoperative motivation for future child bearing, poor couple communication, high conflict levels during decision making, and dominance during decision making by one spouse. Sandlow and colleagues,[59] in a questionnaire study of men before vasectomy, found that patients' anxiety about vasectomy was primarily rooted in fear of pain and fear of the unknown associated with the procedure. Although the patients in this study did not have significant concerns regarding the finality of vasectomy, there was confusion about its reversibility in approximately half of the men. The authors called for preoperative counseling that specifically addressed postoperative expectations and the reversibility of the procedure.

PRIMARY PROGRESSIVE APHASIA

A recent report by Weintraub and colleagues[60] reported an association between vasectomy and PPA, a rare variety of frontotemporal dementia that is associated with a gradual focal decline in language function and relative preservation of memory, cognitive function, and behavioral function during the initial few years of the disease. This 2006 manuscript, published in *Cognitive Behavioral Neurology*, detailed a case-control study comparing 47 men with PPA with 57 controls. Using logistic regression models adjusted for age and education, the rate of vasectomy in patients with PPA was 40% (19 of 47) versus 16% (9 of 57) in the normal controls. This difference in vasectomy rates met statistical significance ($P = .02$). The study also revealed a younger age of PPA onset for patients who had undergone vasectomy (58.79 ± 5.47 versus 62.93 ± 6.77 years; $P = .03$). To date, only one additional manuscript regarding an association between vasectomy and PPA has been published. This study is a case report on a single 68-year-old man with PPA whose clinical condition temporarily improved with a 4-week course of steroid therapy.[61] The authors postulated that their patient's transient clinical improvement, observed in response to a 4-week course of prednisone therapy, supports a possible autoimmune etiology for PPA. Of note, this patient's vasectomy preceded his presentation with PPA by 25 years, and the authors acknowledged several other potential inherent limitations of this case report involving a single patient.

Any causal relationship between vasectomy and PPA is crucial for both individual and public health. Indeed, vasectomies have become exceedingly common over the past several decades, with the prevalence increasing from 3.6% of husbands in 1965 to 15% of husbands in 1995.[62] From 1997 to 2002, approximately 2 million vasectomies were performed in the United States, and approximately 3.5 million women from 15 to 44 years of age were relying on this procedure in their partner as a form of birth control.[63]

Weintraub and colleagues have published numerous manuscripts detailing their work in defining and establishing the diagnosis of the PPA syndrome over the past 20 years. Inspired by one patient's perception regarding his own PPA's pathogenesis, the researchers tested a hypothesis that a correlation exists between vasectomy and PPA. Although the authors have since reported an association between these two entities, the relationship between vasectomy and PPA remains unclear.

In considering the reported association between vasectomy and PPA, it is helpful to use the thoughtful approach investigators used in assessing other putative health risks associated with vasectomy, as has been detailed in this article. Selection bias may have played a role in the observations by Weintraub and colleagues, because men who used the health care system to undergo vasectomy may have been more inclined to use the health care system to seek diagnosis and treatment of a condition, such as PPA. Unaccounted for confounding might also have played a role in the authors' findings. The causal pathway of PPA remains unknown, and potential confounding might exist because the true risk factors for PPA cannot assuredly have been equally distributed between cases and controls. Biologic plausibility is also an important issue to account for when considering a possible association between vasectomy and PPA. The *Cognitive Behavioral Neurology* manuscript hypothesizes that antisperm antibodies may exert effects on the central nervous system, leading to the functional changes seen in PPA. Neuropathologically evaluated brain specimens from patients afflicted by PPA, however, do not typically show evidence of inflammatory infiltrates or other characteristic histologic changes suggestive of an immune-mediated process.

When the initial reports of an association between vasectomy and prostate cancer and vasectomy and testicular cancer surfaced, the World Health Organization concluded, "on the basis of existing biologic and epidemiologic evidence, any causal relationship between vasectomy and the risk of prostate [or testicular] cancer was unlikely and no changes in family planning policies concerning vasectomy are justified."[64] This consensus opinion was again upheld by the World Health Organization in a 1993 review of the literature, following the release of Giovannucci's then news-making reports of an association between vasectomy and prostate cancer.[65] At this time, a similar course of action seems appropriate in regard to the single report of an association between vasectomy and PPA. To date, no multicenter studies have followed, no other single centers have reported similar findings, and no follow-up studies have been published by the authors of the initial report. Given the worldwide benefit of vasectomy, and considering the rare prevalence of PPA and its poorly understood etiology, the burden of proof for causality between vasectomy and PPA should be demonstrated through additional studies before significant alterations in vasectomy practices are undertaken.

SUMMARY

This article reviews the literature regarding the host of broad-ranging health issues that have been previously reported to be associated with vasectomy. These health concerns include the development of cardiovascular disease, testicular cancer, and a variety of immune-complex–mediated disease processes. With follow-up investigation in appropriately designed studies, these initial reported associations have generally been dispelled. Regarding the postulated link between vasectomy and prostate cancer, the bulk of the existing literature does not support a link between these two entities. Several well-designed, population-based studies have revealed a lack of association. Psychologic health can also be negatively impacted in a minority of patients after vasectomy, with investigators recommending that appropriate prevasectomy counseling may help avert many of these problems. Finally, at this time there is a single manuscript reporting an association between vasectomy and PPA. This manuscript has numerous potential intrinsic limitations, including possible bias, confounding, and a lack of clear biologic plausibility. As was undertaken with other health concerns purported to be associated with vasectomy, well-designed follow-up studies are needed to clarify whether there is indeed an association between vasectomy and PPA. To date, no such follow-up studies have been published.

It is certainly important for clinicians to be open-minded as they consider reported correlations between different clinical conditions. As has been exemplified in this article, however, physicians and patients must also be discerning and cautious as they consider reported associations between common procedures (eg, vasectomy) and other health conditions; study design may unintentionally generate statistical associations that are neither scientifically sound nor valid. The use of multiple centers, prospective study design, and minimization of bias and confounding are all strategies that investigators should consider to decrease the likelihood of inauthentic study findings and spurious associations.

REFERENCES

1. Mettlin C, Natarajan N, Huben R. Vasectomy and prostate cancer risk. Am J Epidemiol 1990;132:1056–61.
2. Rosenberg L, Palmer JR, Zauber AG, et al. Vasectomy and the risk of prostate cancer. Am J Epidemiol 1990;132:1051–5.
3. Giovannucci E, Tosteson TD, Speizer FE, et al. A retrospective cohort study of vasectomy and prostate cancer in US men. JAMA 1993;7(269):878–82.
4. Giovannucci E, Ascherio A, Rimm E, et al. A prospective cohort study of vasectomy and prostate cancer in US men. JAMA 1993;7(269):873–7.
5. Strader CH, Weiss NS, Daling JR. Vasectomy and the incidence of testicular cancer. Am J Epidemiol 1988;1(128):56–63.
6. Alexander NJ, Clarkson TB. Vasectomy increases the severity of diet-induced atherosclerosis in *Macaca fascicularis*. Science 1978;4355(201):538–41.
7. Bigazzi P. Immunologic effects of vasectomy in men and experimental animals. Prog Clin Biol Res 1981;70:461–76.
8. Byrne PA, Evans WD, Rajan KT. Does vasectomy predispose to osteoporosis? Br J Urol 1997;4(79):599–601.
9. Alexander NJ, Clarkson TB. Vasectomy increases the severity of diet-induced atherosclerosis in Macaca fascicularis. Science 1978;201(4355):538–41.
10. Clarkson TB, Alexander NJ. Long-term vasectomy: effects on the occurrence and extent of atherosclerosis in rhesus monkeys. J Clin Invest 1980;1(65):15–25.
11. Clarkson TB, Alexander NJ, Morgan TM. Atherosclerosis of cynomolgus monkeys hyper- and hyporesponsive to dietary cholesterol, lack of effect of vasectomy. Arteriosclerosis 1988;8:488–98.
12. Lauersen NH, Muchmore E, Shulman S, et al. Vasectomy and atherosclerosis in *Macaca fascicularis*: new findings in a controversial issue. J Reprod Med 1983;11(28):750–8.
13. Campbell WB, Slack RW, Clifford PC, et al. Vasectomy and atherosclerosis: an association in man? Br J Urol 1983;4(55):430–3.
14. Alexander NJ, Senner JW, Hoch EJ. Evaluation of blood pressure in vasectomized and nonvasectomized men. Int J Epidemiol 1981;3(10):217–22.
15. Goldacre MJ, Holford TR, Vessey MP. Cardiovascular disease and vasectomy: findings from two epidemiologic studies. N Engl J Med 1983;14(308):805–8.
16. Goldacre MJ, Clarke JA, Heasman MA, et al. Follow-up of vasectomy using medical record linkage. Am J Epidemiol 1978;3(108):176–80.
17. Rimm AA, Hoffmann RG, Anderson AJ, et al. The relationship between vasectomy and angiographically determined atherosclerosis in men. Prev Med 1983;2(12):262–73.
18. Rosenberg L, Schwingl PJ, Kaufman DW, et al. The risk of myocardial infarction 10 or more years after vasectomy in men under 55 years of age. Am J Epidemiol 1986;6(123):1049–56.
19. Perrin EB, Woods JS, Namekata T, et al. Long-term effect of vasectomy on coronary heart disease. Am J Public Health 1984;2(74):128–32.
20. Mullooly JP, Wiest WM, Alexander NJ, et al. Vasectomy, serum assays, and coronary heart disease symptoms and risk factors. J Clin Epidemiol 1993;1(46):101–9.
21. Manson JE, Ridker PM, Spelsberg A, et al. Vasectomy and subsequent cardiovascular disease in US physicians. Contraception 1999;3(59):181–6.
22. Giovannucci E, Tosteson TD, Speizer FE, et al. A long-term study of mortality in men who have undergone vasectomy. N Engl J Med 1992;21(326):1392–8.
23. Goldacre MJ, Wotton CJ, Seagroatt V, et al. Cancer and cardiovascular disease after vasectomy: an epidemiological database study. Fertil Steril 2005;5(84):1438–43.
24. Kisker C, Wu K, Culp D, et al. Blood coagulation studies in vasectomy. In: Lepow I, Crozier R, editors. Vasectomy: immunologic and pathophysiologic effects in mammals and man. New York: Academic Press; 1979. p. 105–20.
25. Alexander N, Tung K. Effects of vasectomy in rhesus monkeys. In: Lepow I, Crozier R, editors. Vasectomy: immunologic and pathophysiologic effects in animals and man. New York: Academic Press; 1979. p. 423–55.
26. Nienhuis H, Goldacre M, Seagroatt V, et al. Incidence of disease after vasectomy: a record linkage retrospective cohort study. BMJ 1992;6829(304):743–6.
27. Petitti DB, Klein R, Kipp H, et al. Physiologic measures in men with and without vasectomies. Fertil Steril 1982;3(37):438–40.
28. Linnet L. Clinical immunology of vasectomy and vasovasostomy. Urology 1983;2(22):101–14.
29. Linnet L, Moller NP, Bernth-Petersen P, et al. No increase in arteriolosclerotic retinopathy or activity in tests for circulating immune complexes 5 years after vasectomy. Fertil Steril 1982;6(37):798–806.
30. Witkin SS, Alexander NJ, Frick J. Circulating immune complexes and sperm antibodies following vasectomy in Austrian men. J Clin Lab Immunol 1984;2(14):69–72.
31. Goldacre MJ, Wotton CJ, Seagroatt V, et al. Immune-related disease before and after vasectomy: an

epidemiological database study. Humanit Rep 2007; 5(22):1273–8.

32. Haas G. Male infertility and immunity. In: Lipschultz L, Howards S, editors. Infertility in the male. 2nd edition. Chicago: Mosby-Year Book; 1991. p. 277–96.

33. Rumke P, Hellinga G. Autoantibodies against spermatozoa in sterile men. Am J Clin Pathol 1959;32:357–63.

34. Thornhill JA, Conroy RM, Kelly DG, et al. An evaluation of predisposing factors for testis cancer in Ireland. Eur Urol 1988;6(14):429–33.

35. Cale AR, Farouk M, Prescott RJ, et al. Does vasectomy accelerate testicular tumour? Importance of testicular examinations before and after vasectomy. BMJ 1990;6721(300):370.

36. Jorgensen N, Giwercman A, Hansen SW, et al. Testicular cancer after vasectomy: origin from carcinoma in situ of the testis. Eur J Cancer 1993;7(29A):1062–4.

37. Moller H, Knudsen LB, Lynge E. Risk of testicular cancer after vasectomy: cohort study of over 73,000 men. BMJ 1994;6950(309):295–9.

38. Aetiology of testicular cancer. Association with congenital abnormalities, age at puberty, infertility, and exercise. United Kingdom Testicular Cancer Study Group. BMJ 1994;6941(308):1393–9.

39. Honda GD, Bernstein L, Ross RK, et al. Vasectomy, cigarette smoking, and age at first sexual intercourse as risk factors for prostate cancer in middle-aged men. Br J Cancer 1988;3(57):326–31.

40. Perlman J, Spirtas R, Kelaghan J, et al. Re: vasectomy and the risk of prostate cancer. Am J Epidemiol 1991;134:107.

41. Rosenberg L, Palmer JR, Zauber AG, et al. The relation of vasectomy to the risk of cancer. Am J Epidemiol 1994;5(140):431–8.

42. Schwingl P, Guess HA. Safety and effectiveness of vasectomy. Fertil Steril 2000;73:923–36.

43. Levine RL. Vasectomy and increased risk of prostate cancer. JAMA 1993;270(6):706.

44. DerSimonian R, Clemens J, Spirtas R, et al. Vasectomy and prostate cancer risk: methodological review of the evidence. J Clin Epidemiol 1993;2(46):163–72.

45. Barone MA, Johnson CH, Luick MA, et al. Characteristics of men receiving vasectomies in the United States, 1998–1999. Perspect Sex Reprod Health 2004;1(36):27–33.

46. Piccinino L, Mosher W. Trends in contraceptive use in the United States: 1982–1995. Fam Plann Perspect 1998;1(30):4–46.

47. Howards SS, Peterson HB. Vasectomy and prostate cancer: chance, bias, or a causal relationship? JAMA 1993;7(269):913–4.

48. Sandlow JI, Kreder KJ. A change in practice: current urologic practice in response to reports concerning vasectomy and prostate cancer. Fertil Steril 1996; 66(2):281–4.

49. Cox B, Sneyd MJ, Paul C, et al. Vasectomy and risk of prostate cancer. JAMA 2002;23(287):3110–5.

50. Holt SK, Salinas CA, Stanford JL. Vasectomy and the risk of prostate cancer. J Urol 2008;6(180):2565–7 [discussion: 7–8].

51. Jarow JP, Goluboff ET, Chang TS, et al. Relationship between antisperm antibodies and testicular histologic changes in humans after vasectomy. Urology 1994;4(43):521–4.

52. Raleigh D, O'Donnell L, Southwick GJ, et al. Stereological analysis of the human testis after vasectomy indicates impairment of spermatogenic efficiency with increasing obstructive interval. Fertil Steril 2004;6(81):1595–603.

53. O'Neill DA, McVicar CM, McClure N, et al. Reduced sperm yield from testicular biopsies of vasectomized men is due to increased apoptosis. Fertil Steril 2007; 4(87):834–41.

54. Nicopoullos JD, Gilling-Smith C, Almeida PA, et al. Effect of time since vasectomy and maternal age on intracytoplasmic sperm injection success in men with obstructive azoospermia after vasectomy. Fertil Steril 2004;2(82):367–73.

55. Thonneau P, D'Isle B. Does vasectomy have long-term effects on somatic and psychological health status? Int J Androl 1990;6(13):419–32.

56. Humphrey M, Humphrey H. Vasectomy as a reason for donor insemination. Soc Sci Med 1993;2(37): 263–6.

57. Rogstad KE. The psychological effects of vasectomy. Sex Marital Ther 1996;3(11):265–72.

58. Miller WB, Shain RN, Pasta DJ. The pre- and post-sterilization predictors of poststerilization regret in husbands and wives. J Nerv Ment Dis 1991; 10(179):602–8.

59. Sandlow JI, Westefeld JS, Maples MR, et al. Psychological correlates of vasectomy. Fertil Steril 2001; 3(75):544–8.

60. Weintraub S, Fahey C, Johnson N, et al. Vasectomy in men with primary progressive aphasia. Cogn Behav Neurol 2006;4(19):190–3.

61. Decker DA, Heilman KM. Steroid treatment of primary progressive aphasia. Arch Neurol 2008; 11(65):1533–5.

62. Chandra A. Surgical sterilization in the United States: prevalence and characteristics, 1965–95. Vital Health Stat 23 1998;(20):1–33.

63. Chandra A, Martinez GM, Mosher WD, et al. Fertility, family planning, and reproductive health of U.S. women: data from the 2002 National Survey of Family Growth. Vital Health Stat 23 2005;(25):1–160.

64. Committee WHOS. Vasectomy and cancer. Lancet 1991;338:1586.

65. Farley T, Meirik O, Mehta S, et al. The safety of vasectomy: recent concerns. Bull World Health Organ 1993;71:413–9.

The Law and Vasectomy

Andrew I. Kaplan, Esq*, Jay A. Rappaport, Esq

KEYWORDS

- Malpractice • Wrongful conception • Proximate cause
- Total denial of recovery • Limited recovery
- Full recovery • Offset benefits view
- Common areas of exposure

According to the last annual report of the National Practitioner Data Bank, the central repository of information regarding malpractice payments made on behalf of physicians nationally, during calendar year 2006, 79% of the new reports concerning malpractice payments were physician related, with the median and mean malpractice payment amounts for surgeons totaling $175,000 and $311,965, respectively.[1] Significantly, 3218 malpractice-related payments were made by surgeons in 2006, with the median and mean payouts $145,000 and $252,476, respectively. From 1990 to 2006, almost 64,000 malpractice payouts on behalf of surgeons were reported to the National Practitioner Data Bank.[1]

More pointedly, according to PIAA's 2008 *Risk Management Review* of Urologic Surgery, urologic surgery ranks twelfth in the number of claims reported from 1985 through 2007, among the 26 specialty groups included in the database.[2] The total indemnity paid on behalf of urologists during that time period was $285 million, and also ranked twelfth among the 26 specialty groups reported.[2] In calendar year 2007, over $9 million in indemnity payments for 42 claims in urologic surgery were reported, with an average indemnity payment of $227,838. In all, however, urologic surgery claims, at 2.5%, were a small percentage of claims reported to PIAA in 2007.[2]

Improper performance was the most prevalent medical misadventure claimed in urologic surgery suits. Within that heading, male sterilization procedures ranked fifth among the procedures alleged to have been improperly performed.[2] Of the five most common misadventures resulting in lawsuits (operative procedures on the prostate and seminal vesicles, the bladder, the kidney, the penis, and male sterilization), sterilization was the only one with an average indemnity of less than six figures ($42,143; from 1985–2007). Diagnostic interview, evaluation, and consultation were the "procedures" that resulted in the most claims against urologic surgeons, emphasizing the importance of the information imparted and recorded during the initial patient interaction. Not surprisingly, sterilization procedures ranked first among urologic surgery claims in which the primary injury claimed was emotional.[2]

Medical professionals are certainly familiar with a wide variety of stressors, uncertainties, and hurdles inherent to the practice of medicine, and the practitioner has learned and developed methods and algorithms to deal with them. When physicians are named as defendants in a lawsuit, however, it is akin to entering a foreign land without a passport or an appreciation of the language. It drags practitioners outside of the medical arena and subjects them to forces over which they have little, if any, control and even less knowledge.

Patients who bring such suits, particularly in the realm of "wrongful conception" as a result of a failed or recanalized vasectomy, have their own significant stressors and anxieties. Both sides going forward must understand this fact. It serves no one to engage in characterizations of those who sue, or those who are sued.

This article raises questions and suggests answers as to why the national court system has seen a steady influx of claims alleging practitioners' failure properly to perform vasectomy or ensure sterilization and the manner in which that influx has caused physicians to reassess their methods of practicing medicine in an increasingly litigious environment and make the appropriate and necessary accommodations. Through their experiences

Aaronson, Rappaport, Feinstein & Deutsch, LLP, 757 Third Avenue, New York, NY 10017, USA
* Corresponding author.
E-mail address: aikaplan@arfdlaw.com (A.I. Kaplan).

Urol Clin N Am 36 (2009) 347–357
doi:10.1016/j.ucl.2009.05.002

as medical malpractice litigators and through the analysis of reported cases, national jury verdicts, and insurance claims made and paid in lawsuits arising from claims regarding the performance of vasectomy, the authors hope to enlighten the reader as to the legal theories and hurdles applicable to such claims and the medical theories most often elucidated and litigated by the patients who bring them. At the conclusion of this article the authors offer suggestions as to the manner in which the practitioner may be proactive in both preventing and defending exposure to malpractice litigation.

WHAT IS MALPRACTICE?

The authors have always found it instructive, whether discussing the matter with physicians or laypersons, to educate the listener as to the charge delivered by the Court to the average jury member sitting in judgment in a medical malpractice action, just before commencing deliberation. Malpractice, as defined by the *Pattern Jury Instructions*, from whence the Court derives its ultimate charge to the jury, reads as follows (**Box 1**):

Malpractice litigation is a form of tort, or civil (as opposed to criminal), litigation wherein a patient, termed the "plaintiff," brings the action accusing a physician, the defendant, of a civil wrong. That civil wrong is negligence: failure to act as a "reasonable person" or to adhere to a particular standard of care. Negligence by a professional is termed "malpractice," and by a physician or hospital "medical malpractice." The burden of proving every essential element that constitutes malpractice in any given case remains with the patient from institution of the proceeding until verdict is rendered and judgment entered.

In medical malpractice litigation, the standard of care arises from the physician's responsibility to possess and apply that reasonable degree of skill, learning, and ability ordinarily possessed by physicians within the community in which he or she practices. The standard of care within the community in which the defendant practices changes on a case-by-case basis, because prior trial court decisions in similar actions have no precedential or binding effect. There is no set standard of care adherent to the performance of vasectomy, nor could there be one, irrespective of the existence of published guidelines by any number of urologic associations. Although persuasive evidence of a practitioner's breach from what is considered accepted protocol in the urologic community, absent concession that they are "authoritative" or "controlling," guidelines are

---

Box 1
PJI 2:150: malpractice–physician

Malpractice is professional negligence and medical malpractice is the negligence of a doctor. Negligence is the failure to use reasonable care under the circumstances, doing something that a reasonably prudent doctor would not do under the circumstances, or failing to do something that a reasonably prudent doctor would do under the circumstances. It is a deviation or departure from accepted practice.

A doctor who renders medical service to a patient is obligated to have that reasonable degree of knowledge and skill that is expected of an average specialist who (performs, provides) that (operation, treatment, medical service) in the medical community in which the doctor practices.

The law recognizes that there are differences in the abilities of doctors, just as there are differences in the abilities of people engaged in other activities. To practice medicine a doctor is not required to have the extraordinary knowledge and ability that belongs to a few doctors of exceptional ability. However every doctor is required to keep reasonably informed of new developments in (his, her) field and to practice (medicine, surgery) in accordance with approved methods and means of treatment in general use. A doctor must also use his or her best judgment and whatever superior knowledge and skill (he, she) possesses, even if the knowledge and skill exceeds that possessed by the average specialist in the medical community where the doctor practices.

By undertaking to perform a medical service, a doctor does not guarantee a good result. The fact that there was a bad result to the patient, by itself, does not make the doctor liable. The doctor is liable only if (he, she) was negligent. Whether the doctor was negligent is to be decided on the basis of the facts and conditions existing at the time of the claimed negligence.

A doctor is not liable for an error in judgment if (he, she) does what (he, she) decides is best after careful evaluation if it is a judgment that a reasonably prudent doctor could have made under the circumstances.

If the doctor is negligent, that is, lacks the skill or knowledge required of (him, her) in providing a medical service, or fails to use reasonable care in providing the service, or fails to exercise his or her best judgment, and such failure is a substantial factor in causing harm to the patient, then the doctor is responsible for the injury or harm caused.

just that, guidelines. Deviation from them is not, standing alone, evidence of per se negligence. In each individual situation it is the duty of the fact-finder (the jury) and occasionally of the appellate courts, in situations where the jury's decision is inconsistent with the facts or the law presented, to determine just what the applicable standard of care is in any given situation and to determine whether that standard was met by the defendant physician.

To establish a claim for civil negligence, there must first be proof of a duty owed (a "physician-patient relationship"). That relationship arises any time a physician undertakes to diagnose or treat urologic conditions, whether it be during examination within the confines of the office, operating in a hospital or ambulatory care facility, rendering advice over the telephone to one's own patient, or while on call for a colleague.

Once it has been established that a duty to render appropriate care exists, the next prong in establishing a claim for medical malpractice lies in proving a breach of that duty (commonly defined as a departure or deviation from good and accepted practice or care). Whether or not the physician breached is a determination made by the jury based on the medical evidence in the case and the testimony of the witnesses. More often than not, it is the testimony and the credibility of the expert witnesses in the case on the subjects of standard of care in the community and whether the particular practitioner on trial adhered to or departed from that standard that influences a jury's decision. Those experts are subject to cross-examination by opposing counsel, not only on the medical testimony given on the stand but on their qualifications, credibility, and in the face of inconsistent sworn testimony they may have given previously on similar topics in other courts of law.

Medical treatises or guidelines applicable to the period of treatment at issue, and the defendant's own prior testimony, publications, and office protocols, may also come into play in the jury's analysis. Most courts adhere to the common rule that a text or treatise must first be acknowledged as authoritative in the field before it may be read to the jury, but once acknowledged as such it may be used to establish that the defendant practitioner deviated from the authoritative standards as set forth within the publication and committed malpractice.

Most attorneys who select juries on behalf of patients tell those juries that they are not claiming that the practitioner acted or failed to act intentionally, or that they are "bad" doctors. Instead, they allege one act or series of acts of malpractice as isolated incidents of breach of care in a longer history of good practice. Without a "bad result," meaning without injury, there is no case, but every jury is charged that a bad result, in and of itself, is not evidence of malpractice. It is not the result that legally determines if there was negligence. Practically speaking, however, a jury faced with a bad result undoubtedly considers that result in the exercise of deliberation.

An error in medical judgment is not evidence of malpractice. In context, the use of the word "judgment" here has a specific meaning. Judgment comes into play in the arena of malpractice litigation where, and only where, there are two or more ways for a physician to approach a situation. If there are two ways to deal with the situation, each acceptable in the medical community, the choice by the physician of the one over the other is the exercise of judgment, and if exercised appropriately the physician can be defended even if the chosen treatment failed.

Many a practitioner has attempted to defend an allegation of malpractice by asserting that an exercise of judgment cannot constitute negligence, and many a tribunal has allowed the pursuit of just such a defense. In reality, however, almost every action involving a physician's decision making as it pertained to a patient could conceivably be defended as such, and so the courts have attempted to limit the defense of "judgment" to those situations where the practitioner had two very real and very acceptable treatment options available and chose one over the other to the unfortunate but unpredictable detriment of the patient.

In that regard, jurors are cautioned against casting their judgment on the defendant physician based on outcome, but rather are directed to consider what the physician had in front of him or her at the time care was rendered and decisions made. The reason for this directive is that in hindsight almost all are correct.

The third and most essential prong in establishing medical malpractice is causation. It must be shown that the practitioner's action or inaction was the competent, or primary, producing cause of injury to the patient. The burden is on the patient to prove that, more likely than not, earlier or alternative diagnosis or treatment would have positively affected outcome. It is not the patient's burden to establish that appropriate care would have resulted in some guaranteed result (although in some situations that is the very allegation made, particularly when it comes to the subject of "permanent sterilization"). Rather, it is enough to establish that it would have impacted the quality and duration of life to the patient's benefit. So significant is the subject of causation that it maintains its own pattern jury instruction. Proximate cause is defined in the *Pattern Jury Instructions* as follows (**Box 2**):

Acknowledging that a delay in diagnosis (even a negligent delay) may not affect the patient's ultimate outcome, or that surgical "error" or postoperative management may not cause or contribute to the specific injury claimed, the law interposes the evidentiary requirement of "proximate cause" on plaintiffs seeking monetary damages in medical malpractice cases. Technically, if a physician's negligence did not cause harm, the patient should be unable to make out what is known as a "prima facie," or sufficient on its face, case of medical malpractice that survives dismissal at the close of plaintiff's evidence rather than reaches the deliberation of the jury. In reality, however, rare is the action in which medical negligence is proved yet the claim dismissed by Court or jury. As discussed further, the public perceives that accurate diagnosis and treatment alters outcome, and the public is often unwilling to forgive the practitioner who has breached the standard of care or accept that "it didn't make a difference."

The final prong in establishing a claim of medical malpractice is that the patient must have sustained an actual injury as a result of the practitioner's malpractice to obtain reward for final damages. Although punitive or punishment damage awards are rare, juries are instructed that under the appropriate circumstances they can award noneconomic damages for pain and suffering and loss of consortium or society (an award made for harm to a close relationship, such as with a spouse or child). It is common for a patient's spouse to be named as coplaintiff in a malpractice action, to seek redress for loss of society, comfort, and companionship because of the injuries alleged, and to obtain remuneration in significant amounts in those cases wherein a jury determines that plaintiffs have proved their claims.

Economic damages, such as loss of earnings incurred to date and in the future, medical costs, rehabilitation and therapy costs, and out-of-pocket expenses for goods and services can be granted and often constitute a hefty portion of the fees awarded. Cases involving allegations of wrongful conception are controversial, and although few jurisdictions award damages consistent with the cost of raising a healthy but "unwanted" child, most offer both spouses avenue to pursue compensatory damages for injuries inflicted (discussed later).

As a caveat, although the burden of proof in all cases rests on the party asserting the claim, the defense must prove those issues raised by the defense, which are deemed "affirmative defenses," and which must be set forth in the initial answer to the complaint. Perhaps the most significant of these affirmative defenses in the realm of vasectomy litigation is termed "culpable conduct," or more correctly, "comparative negligence," which is conduct by the patient that caused or contributed to their own damages and may reduce the ultimate verdict by the percentage of that culpability.

In the area of vasectomy litigation, this usually means that the patient did not follow an instruction that, if followed, would have improved his outcome or prognosis. Quite frequently it involves ignorance of admonitions to submit semen samples for analysis or to avoid unprotected sexual relations until a specified number of postoperative fertility studies can be performed, but it can be as simple as ignoring a surgeon's warnings regarding postoperative hygiene, which contributes to wound breakdown, poor healing, and infection. Because in many instances in this area of litigation the patient has sought a "guaranteed" means of sterilization for personal, economic, or even emotional reasons, this defense is one approached with care and trepidation. The patient's attorney attempts to portray the defense and the doctor as "blaming the patient." To be effective, such a defense must not only be medically valid, but the basis for the defense must be well documented in the defendant physician's records and supported by the records of other nonparty treating practitioners, such as the family physician.

Who Sues Whom and Why?

It has been the author's experience that almost any surgeon with a busy practice invariably ends up on the "wrong side" of a malpractice suit. That is not to suggest that all practitioners find themselves defendants in a lawsuit, or that only those with a high-volume practice get sued. But more often than not, today's practitioner faces

---

Box 2
PJI 2:70: proximate cause–in general

An act or omission is regarded as a cause of an injury if it was a substantial factor in bringing about the injury, that is, if it had such an effect in producing the injury that reasonable people would regard it as a cause of the injury. There may be more than one cause of an injury, but to be substantial, it cannot be slight or trivial. You may, however, decide that a cause is substantial even if you assign a relatively small percentage to it.

the service of a summons and complaint, or at least the specter of a malpractice claim.

Research reveals that a significant percentage of malpractice lawsuits involving the performance of vasectomy sound in "wrongful conception" or "wrongful pregnancy," an action brought by the parents of a healthy, but unexpected, unplanned, or unwanted child for alleged negligence leading to conception or pregnancy. The simple fact of the matter, however, is that every interaction with a patient in this litigious society is rife with the potential for a malpractice claim. The referral, the initial intake, the history and physical examination, and the consent to surgery are all potential avenues of omission or commission that can give strength or support to a patient's claim of surgical negligence. The actual physical performance of surgery itself, replete with risks and complications, is the focal point of many a malpractice claim sounding in vasectomy. Postoperative evaluation, recommendation, and, in particular, fertility testing, however, can be equally as perilous.

With that in mind, the initial consultative visit takes on increased importance and must be approached with the patient's anxiety in mind. As with any legal situation, documentation is the key, but the creation of a physician-patient relationship and particularly the ephemeral forging of trust can decrease the risk of subsequent exposure. Time should be taken to answer any and all patient questions and those questions should be encouraged. The procedure itself should be discussed along with risks, potential complications, and any contraindications. If a patient is willing to bring his spouse or partner along for the visit, all the better, because a second witness to a detailed conversation regarding what to expect affords the attorney more opportunity to obtain helpful testimony should the case proceed to deposition.

From a litigation perspective, that consultative visit, as routine as it may be, warrants a clear, concise progress note in the patient's chart. Simply writing "initial consultation," although expedient and likely illustrative to the practitioner, leaves little to support the extent and thoroughness of the conversation with the patient on that date. Better at least to outline the fact that risks, complications, and the nature of the procedure were discussed (without necessarily outlining each and every risk and complication, because invariably one will arise that has been omitted, and will afford opposing counsel ammunition to argue it was never discussed or contemplated, but its disclosure was warranted).

Assuming time is taken to discuss the nature of the procedure and brochures are given, or models or illustrations used, documentation of this in the initial progress note is helpful. Often, incredulous testimony can be stretched to the breaking point in the face of such specificity, particularly the use of demonstrative evidence. If the patient agrees to undergo the procedure at this initial visit, the consent forms should be signed and copies placed in the patient's chart, accurately dated, and witnessed. If the physician or practitioner can take the extra step of having the patient execute a consent form, verifying that the patient was encouraged to ask any questions that came to mind and that all questions were answered to the patient's satisfaction, all the better.

If the procedure itself was discussed at the initial consultation, clear instructions in printed form should be given to the patient for both preoperative and postoperative procedures. The patient should be told in detail what he needs to do to prepare for the surgery and what he can expect postoperatively. The concepts of rest, limited activities, bathing or swimming, sexual intercourse, and even the need to ejaculate postoperatively to clear the sperm ducts should be discussed and documented with the patient signing off on receipt of both preoperative and postoperative instructions. Carbons of those executed acknowledgments should be made part of the patient's chart or scanned into the computer file.

Research and experience reveal that a cause of action sounding in lack of informed consent (the alleged failure to adequately warn or instruct the patient as to the potential risks, benefits, and alternatives of the planned procedure, combined with the plaintiff's claim that had he been made aware of those potential pitfalls, no matter how remote, he would have deferred surgery or sought alternative care) is invariably part and parcel of a patient's claim. Careful, reasonable documentation of those conversations is the most effective weapon in the physician's arsenal.

By way of illustration, consider the 1996 California case of *Cole v. Korcek*, JVR No. 183,897 (Cal.Superior), 1996 WL 643,370. A husband and wife with two daughters sued for wrongful conception after the patient underwent vasectomy and his wife subsequently gave birth to their third child. They contended they could not afford the cost of another child and that they drove vintage 1969 Mustangs and could not equip the vehicles for five people. The plaintiffs insisted that the defendant physician advised them that a single postoperative semen sample was negative, and that this was sufficient to permit them to engage in unprotected intercourse. The plaintiff added a cause of action for lack of informed consent, contending he would not have elected to undergo the vasectomy if he had been made aware of the failure rates.

Fortunately for the defendant physician, his chart accurately reflected his admonition that the semen sample was positive and that the patient was advised to continue to use protective measures during intercourse. A follow-up letter was sent and a copy annexed to the chart reminding the patient to bring another semen sample to the office for testing. The jury accepted that it was the sole responsibility of the patient to submit specimens for analysis, and rejected the consent claim, finding that no reasonable person who wished to undergo sterilization would refuse based on the miniscule failure rate. A verdict in favor of the defense was awarded.

Although most vasectomy-related lawsuits surround wrongful conception, the other more routine complications of vasectomy should be discussed, and do occasionally form the basis of claims. Patients have brought suits for infection, sperm granuloma, sperm congestion, or the development of sperm antibodies. Lawsuits have been commenced as a result of chronic testicular pain, which lasts long-term after vasectomy, even though these are published and accepted complications of the procedure. Claims sounding in informed consent are bolstered by the plaintiff's attestation that had he known or been made aware of these complications, he would have opted not to have surgery.

In cases involving vasectomy, because of the reluctance and anxiety involved (not to mention the sensitive anatomy) jurors might be more apt to accept that a patient would have deferred an undesirable and elective procedure based on the knowledge of untoward complications than in cases, for example, sounding in the need to remove potentially metastatic tumors or repair obstructed bowel. By the same token, however, research and experience reflect that in the face of well-documented, contemporaneous disclosure of the risks and potential complications to a patient who appreciates them, jurors are inclined to take a "you knew what you were getting yourself into" demeanor in the courtroom.

Consider the recent Texas case of *Holt v. Frankel*, 2007 WL 4,623,848, (Collin Cty, Texas, 2007). The evening after his vasectomy, the patient called the defendant physician to complain of pain, swelling, and a discolored scrotum. After being told his symptoms were "normal" for postoperative day number 1, the patient called back 2 days later to reiterate his complaints and was again told not to worry. Two days later he wound up in a local hospital after his scrotum swelled to twice its normal size and a testicular ultrasound revealed no blood flow to the left testicle. It was removed

the following morning. The patient sued for medical expenses, pain and suffering, mental anguish, and loss of body member and disfigurement, alleging the physician was negligent in failing to warn of the dangers of vasectomy, failing properly and timely to treat the patient, and failing to recognize the symptoms as serious complications of the surgery. His wife sued to recover damages for her loss of consortium and household services.

The defendant contended that there was no evidence of when the loss of blood flow occurred and that it likely was an acute event on the day of hospitalization. He further contended that his records accurately reflected a thorough consent conversation, including the patient's understanding of the risks of bleeding and infection and damage to adjacent organs, inclusive of the patient's scrotum and testes. The jury found for the defendant. It seems that in this instance, the patient strained his own credibility by insisting he had never been instructed by the defendant in the dangers of vasectomy, particularly when the chart suggested otherwise. This led the jury to decide the ever crucial credibility battle in favor of the physician, and forgive his theoretical delay in diagnosis.

WRONGFUL CONCEPTION

Wrongful conception is an action brought by the parents of a normal, healthy, but unplanned child to recover damages for allegedly causing a conception or pregnancy when the couple had sought the physician's assistance in avoiding such occurrence. Today, wrongful conception is a widely accepted cause of action. Compensation for child-rearing expenses for the birth of a healthy child is the most controversial aspect of damage awards. Most courts today still refuse to award damages for the full cost of these child-rearing expenses. The compensation theories used by courts can be grouped into four categories: (1) total denial of recovery, (2) limited recovery, (3) full recovery, and (4) offset benefits (**Box 3**).

Total Denial of Recovery

Until 20 years ago, when the incidence of prenatal torts increased, the total denial of recovery approach was the predominant approach used by courts in wrongful conception actions. Currently, only Kansas and Nevada still adhere to this approach, neither recognizing the tort nor awarding damages in wrongful conception claims. The supreme courts of these two states rely on the old common law rationale used to deny this cause of action: that the birth of a healthy child is not a harm. As a matter of public

Box 3
State high courts' or federal courts' decisions on wrongful life according to state

Recognizing and upholding claims for wrongful conception (most involving healthy children)

Alabama, Alaska, Arizona, Arkansas, Connecticut, District of Columbia, Florida, Georgia, Illinois, Indiana, Kansas, Louisiana, Maine, Maryland, Massachusetts, Minnesota, Missouri, New Hampshire, New Mexico, North Carolina, Ohio, Oregon, Pennsylvania, Rhode Island, Tennessee, Utah, Vermont, Virginia, Washington, West Virginia, Wisconsin, Wyoming

Upholding claims in cases involving children with impairments

Connecticut (orthopedic abnormality); Florida (congenital defects); Georgia (club foot);

Louisiana (albinism); North Carolina (genetic defect); Ohio (birth defect); Pennsylvania (neurofibromatosis)

States also including costs of rearing healthy child in full

New Mexico, Oregon, Washington

States allowing costs of rearing healthy child but offset by benefits of rearing child

Arizona, Connecticut, Maryland, Massachusetts, Minnesota

Denying recovery because it was not a foreseeable consequence of negligent sterilization

Ohio, Louisiana

Birth impairment considered when assessing other damages but not allowing costs of child rearing

Florida, Georgia, Pennsylvania

Also accepting costs of child rearing

North Carolina

Case-by-case approach

Connecticut

Rejecting claims for wrongful conception

Iowa (failed abortion); Kentucky; New York; Oklahoma; Texas (last three for negligent sterilization, all involving healthy children)

Including both healthy children and those born with congenital impairments

Texas

Healthy children only

New York, Oklahoma, Kentucky, Nevada

No law

California; Colorado; Delaware; Hawaii (decision but only addressed civil procedure issues, not underlying action); Idaho; Michigan; Mississippi; Montana; Nebraska; New Jersey; North Dakota; South Carolina; South Dakota

policy, these courts rule that there is no cause of action for wrongful conception.

For example, in 1986, the Nevada Supreme Court, in *Szekeres v. Robinson*, declined to award any damages for wrongful conception, and held that such cases were not to be analyzed under a negligence scheme. The *Szekeres* court found that even if the doctor's negligent or careless conduct contributed to the birth of a child, it does not rise to a tort liability in negligence because the birth of a healthy baby was not a legally compensable damage. Nevertheless,

the court stated that its denial of tort liability did not mean that plaintiffs could not recover under a breach of contract claim. According to the court, the damages in a breach of contract claim are limited to the cost of medical, surgical, and hospital care associated with the failed surgery.

Limited Recovery

The second approach to damages in wrongful conception case is the limited recovery view. This approach is the one espoused by most jurisdictions in the United States. The Courts using this method allow damages for harm that is the direct result of the physician's negligence but preclude recovery for child-rearing expenses. According to these courts, a parent should not be awarded the costs of child rearing because such damages are too speculative. These courts also reason that (1) the benefits of a healthy child outweigh any economic loss, (2) child-rearing expenses are disproportionate to the doctor's culpability, and (3) there are devastating psychologic effects when a child later finds out he or she was unwanted and that someone else is paying to rear him or her. In declining to award child-rearing expenses, these courts also are concerned with the possible increase in fraudulent claims and the difficulty in drawing a line to stop the physician's liability. These courts do not honor a patient's request to be compensated for the costs of child rearing, but find that other damages, such as medical expenses, loss of consortium, emotional distress, loss of wages, and pain and suffering, are appropriate.

Full Recovery

The third approach to awarding damages in wrongful conception cases is full recovery. The jurisdictions applying this view allow recovery for all damages that are incidental to the pregnancy, including child-rearing expenses. Some of these courts have reasoned that it is not speculative to award these costs because juries are accustomed to calculating these costs in other types of tort actions. According to these courts, public policy considerations do not preclude the recovery of child-rearing and education expenses because even the birth of a healthy child imposes certain costs on parents, costs they had sought to avoid. Furthermore, some courts have stated that public policy compels recovery of child-rearing damages to protect the right to family planning.

In 1990, for example, the Supreme Court of Wisconsin, in *Marciniak v. Lundborg*, held that the parents of a healthy child may recover damages, including child-rearing expenses, from a physician who negligently performed a sterilization procedure. The court found that these costs should not be offset by the benefits conferred on the parents by the presence of a healthy child in their lives.

In finding the physician negligent, the *Marciniak* court explained that no public policy considerations prevented the recognition of liability. The court stated that traditional principles of tort liability should apply and a wrongdoer must compensate those who are injured by his or her negligence. According to the Court, child-rearing costs are not speculative because similar types of costs are awarded in numerous other types of cases, such as wrongful death cases. Moreover, these damages are not out of proportion to the doctor's culpability because they are foreseeable. Additionally, public policy does not immunize defendants from liability merely because the damages are substantial. The Court reasoned that awarding child-rearing damages to the parents would not psychologically damage the child, but rather it would alleviate the family's economic burdens and add to the well-being of the child. Finally, the *Marciniak* court reasoned that it would not be equitable to force on the parents the costs of raising a child when they sought precisely to avoid those costs.

The Offset Benefits View

The fourth approach to damages in wrongful conception cases is referred to as the "offset benefits view." Courts using this method reject the view that, as a matter of law, child-rearing expenses are not recoverable. These courts, however, do not go as far as full recovery because they hold that the child-rearing damages should be offset by the benefit the parents receive from having a healthy child. These courts draw this principle from Section 920 of the *Restatement (Second) of Torts*, which states that when a defendant's tortuous act causes harm to the plaintiff but also confers a benefit, such benefit should be considered in mitigation of damages to the extent it is equitable. Jurisdictions using this approach allow the jury to decide when child-rearing costs exceed the benefits, and allow plaintiffs to recover the difference between the costs and the benefit. Some courts have refined this process and take into account the plaintiff's motivation for seeking the sterilization procedure. Those courts that take the parents' motivation into account are more likely to allow recovery for the costs of child-rearing if the primary motivation was financial. If the parents seek sterilization, however, for eugenic reasons (eg, avoidance of a genetic defect), or out of concern for the mother's health, then recovery for these costs is less justified.

In 1983, the Supreme Court of Arizona, in *University of Arizona Health Sciences Center v. Superior Court*, adopted the offset benefits view and held that the benefits of an unplanned but healthy child may be weighed against any pecuniary and nonpecuniary damages in determining plaintiffs' recovery in a wrongful conception case. The *University of Arizona* court found that a health care provider operating a teaching hospital could be liable for negligently performing a vasectomy. The plaintiffs were a husband and wife, who after having three children decided not to have any more children. The husband and wife decided that a vasectomy was the best means of contraception for them. After the husband underwent the vasectomy operation, the wife became pregnant and delivered a healthy child. Subsequently, the husband and wife sued the doctor and his employer, the teaching hospital, seeking damages including child-rearing expenses.

The *University of Arizona* court, after discussing the approaches taken by courts throughout the country, reasoned that child-rearing damages are compensable but should be offset by the benefits of the parent-child relationship. The court recognized that the birth of a healthy child is not always a benefit, depending on the reasons behind the parents' decision not to have another child. Although in some cases a family can adjust to the birth of a child they were not expecting, in other cases the birth of an unplanned child can cause serious emotional and economic problems to the parents.

The court reasoned that the costs of child-rearing should be offset by the pecuniary and nonpecuniary benefits conferred on the parents according to the particular circumstances of the case. For example, the court suggested that such factors as family size, family income, age of the parents, and marital status be taken into account when calculating the benefit to the parents. According to the court, the offset benefits approach allows the jury certain flexibility in determining which persons have suffered more or gained more as a result of the birth of a healthy child. The court also reasoned that denying compensation for child-rearing expenses deviates from one of the basic principles of tort law: that a wrongdoer is held liable for all damages that he or she caused and all costs that the victim sustains as a result of the wrong. The court determined that this case-by-case adjudication in determining child-rearing damages, despite its inevitable variations, provides the most accurate method in computing damages in wrongful conception cases.

Common Areas of Exposure

Courts in some jurisdictions allow recovery for the mother's emotional distress associated with an unplanned or unwanted pregnancy and delivery, secondary to a "failed sterilization." For example, in *Custodio v. Bower* 251 Cal. App 2d 303 (1967), the California Appellate Division held that if the parents could show physical complications and mental, physical, and nervous pain and suffering that the sterilization procedure was designed to

prevent, they should be able to recover. The Court held that mental suffering attendant to an unexpected pregnancy because of the complications both physical and financial that might or might not result and those that did result were all foreseeable consequences of a failure of sterilization.

Research reflects that the lion's share of vasectomy lawsuits sounding in wrongful conception involve allegations of negligence in the recommendation or postoperative performance of semen analysis. In *Johnston v. Elkins*, a Kansas case, the defendant surgeon told the patient 1 month after vasectomy that he was sterile based on his semen sample. Although the guidelines of the health plan of which the surgeon was an agent and employee called for two postoperative semen examinations before a determination of the success of a vasectomy could be made, the surgeon told the patient he only needed one test. Relying on this advice, the family stopped using contraceptives, the mother became pregnant, and a follow-up examination indicated the presence of sperm in the father's semen. Although the court disallowed recovery for emotional damages, it permitted recovery for the expense of the unsuccessful vasectomy; the father's pain and suffering; the cost of prenatal care, delivery, and the mother's subsequent tubal ligation; and loss of consortium for the applicable time period.

Likewise, in *Garrison v. Foy*, an Indiana case, and *Owens v. Foote*, a case venued in Tennessee, the courts did not permit recovery for the emotional anguish of delivering a deformed child subsequent to negligent vasectomy, or the unexpected costs of raising a brain-damaged child, although recovery was permitted for those damages arising from the unsuccessful sterilization and resultant pregnancy. At perhaps the extreme end of the analysis is the Federal case of *Ostergard v. US*, 677 F Supp 1259 (1987), where the practitioner's advice to the patient to "go home and have fun," was deemed a misrepresentation of the patient's sterility and resulted in the fathering of an unexpected and unwanted child. Needless to say, the authors are constrained to counsel against such glib pronouncements, at least without the benefit of concretely supportive semen analysis.

Erroneously assuming that a sufficient amount of time has passed since vasectomy to ensure sterility, without repeating semen analysis, is a fact pattern that has repeated itself in the malpractice annals. So, too, are claims wherein the practitioner essentially "loses track" of the patient, and although multiple postoperative semen samples are analyzed, they never actually fall below the minimum count generally considered necessary for fertility. These cases are often defended by pointing out the patient's responsibility to submit samples until they are ensured of infertility, but can be rather easily avoided with careful attention to detail and an ingrained office protocol for the ensurance of sterility.

Defendants in wrongful conception or wrongful birth cases may seek to deny culpability on the basis that the plaintiff consented to the treatment or the procedure. Although a court may examine a consent document to see whether it addresses the conduct at issue, generally courts have found that such documents do not remove or reduce a professional's liability resulting from negligent conduct, such as medical malpractice. Courts have determined that, as a matter of public policy, professionals should not be able to protect themselves from their own negligence, as opposed to any inherent risks of a procedure or condition, through disclaimers or waivers that attempt to transfer the risks to patients or nonprofessionals. Some courts have also noted that patients are not in an equal bargaining position with a medical professional and it is unfair to enforce a waiver for that reason. The extent to which language in signed consent forms that outline risks may limit professional exposure is unclear, particularly because state laws and courts vary regarding the degree to which they take such forms into account.

WHAT IS A PHYSICIAN TO DO?

It is imperative for all physicians to be aware that the most important requirement of effective defense in litigation is documentation. If a fact, finding, or recommendation is not documented, the issue of its existence becomes almost purely one of credibility, a contest between the healthy physician against the individual, frequently injured, patient. In context, it is important to realize that the physician has many patients, and has seen many of them between the incidents complained of and the lawsuit. The patient, however, has one thing to recall: his own treatment.

This is not to say the patient's recall is at all times accurate, or that the physician's is not. Common sense dictates that in this area the patient has an advantage, however, which can be reduced or removed by appropriate, thorough documentation. It is not really enough to say, "I always do it." If "it" is important enough to "always do," it is important enough to "always document."

Documentation of a pertinent finding or recommendation and the fact that it has been conveyed to the patient or appropriate physician serves not only contemporaneously to establish the nature and purpose of treatment recommended and

given, but to aid in the practitioner's legal defense months or years down the road, when memories have faded or become biased by health problems, and credibility between the parties is at issue.

Jurors have a natural inclination to accept what is written in a medical record as truth, or to at least provide the documented medical chart with the preferential inference of accuracy. In this way, communication and documentation truly go hand in hand. The passage of time, the backdrop of litigation, the sympathy afforded an injured patient or his family, and the suspicion of a physician's presumed self-interest can all be countered by a medical record replete with pertinent findings and recommendations entered contemporaneously with treatment, long before the prospect of litigation was ever entertained.

The practitioner and counsel are always advantaged by the maintenance of a complete chart. By complete, is meant one that contains all notes by the physician, all reports received, and all memoranda that have to do with follow-up. Telephone messages received should be acknowledged in the chart (stapled to a page is always good), and the response to them documented.

In addition to documenting all recommendations, documenting thought process (the diagnoses and tests considered and ruled out, as well as why) provides credible explanations of the judgment applied to potential jurors down the road. Documenting follow-up on any and all recommendations is imperative. On the next visit, a follow-up note can, and should, be generated. Did the patient comply? If not, why not, and if so, when? Again, the testimony that "I always ask" is not as effective as a note documenting that the question was asked and a response received.

Some patients do not return after a recommendation for treatment or consult is made. Because most of these recommendations are or should be timed (ie, motility testing "next week"), a follow-up system that accounts for the receipt of an appropriate report or consult note is helpful in countering the subtle, and sometimes not so subtle, indication by the patient's attorney that the physician in question did not care, or worse, abandoned the patient. These allegations are based on the unspoken but real supposition that in medical matters patients have given up the skills and knowledge they use in their everyday lives, and have become dependent on the special skills of others. Because most jurors are also patients, this argument holds weight and can sway opinion. Accurate documentation of a patient's reluctance to follow recommendations, pursue treatment, or keep appointments can help to counter the allegation that any delay or error was necessarily occasioned by the physician.

The courtroom is not a theater or a sports arena. There are, indeed, both theatrical and sports analogies used in the description and practice of the litigation process, but these analogies are often suspect. Using them is, however, helpful in developing the appropriate litigation mindset.

Language is important to all of us, and in the courtroom it is particularly important. It takes a back seat in the context of litigation, however, to attitude. This is why physicians are directed to consider themselves as fact witnesses, not defendants, and that they are not to defend their case, which is the responsibility and province of counsel. The reasons for this are multifactorial. First, once such words as "defense" are being used, one is in the realm of the lawyer, not the realm of the doctor. The simple reality is that the defense of any case is the attorney's job, whereas the careful and truthful rendition of the facts and circumstances surrounding the incidents in question is the witness' job, be that witness a nonparty or the defendant.

It must be understood that sympathy is the unacknowledged, impermissible (the court advises the jury not to use sympathy in its determinations) factor that must be recognized and controlled when possible. The physician defendant does not engender sympathy in the face of the injured parties. Any attitude other than professional commitment and concern work against the physician as a witness.

This does not mean that true sincerity, or caring, cannot be shown. It is antagonism toward the process, or the participants, that must be avoided. Although the sporting arena analogy, with its theme of two sides in competition, is comparable, it is often, ultimately, counterproductive. Similarly, the "courtroom as theater" analogy distracts. Jurors, increasingly more sophisticated and litigation savvy, detect actors and disregard them. Conversely they respond to a knowledgeable professional who presents without obvious ego, calmly indicating facts and opinions that bolster the reality of the defense.

Communication is the key element in establishing credibility and rapport with a patient and in gaining a patient's trust. In the cases that the authors have litigated either at the time of deposition or at trial, the patient sets forth the basis for bringing suit: "He did not tell me a thing." "She ignored my complaints." "He showed no compassion." "He never told me I needed a follow-up appointment." "I was never told of bleeding," or "pain" or "recanalization" or "failure." The list is endless but it always centers on the patient's underlying mistrust of the physician for failing to convey simply and accurately pertinent findings and recommendations in a professional and timely manner.

As cliché as it may seem, the "relationship" between physician and patient is often a key determining factor in whether or not a patient chooses to pursue legal remedy against a physician, irrespective of whether or not a departure from appropriate care occurred. The way the patient views his relationship with the physician matters.

In terms of preventing litigation, the role of physician as compassionate caregiver should not be underestimated. Reality informs us, however, that even thoughtful physicians who communicate well can be and are sued. As verdict awards increase, even the most compassionate of caregivers may ultimately find themselves in a courtroom. It is the hope of the authors that they will be well prepared.

REFERENCES

1. National Practitioner Data Bank 2006 Annual Report.
2. PIAA Risk Management Review. 2008 Edition Urologic Surgery.

History of Vasectomy Reversal

Howard H. Kim, MD[a,b,c], Marc Goldstein, MD, FACS[a,b,c],*

KEYWORDS
- Vasectomy reversal • Vasovasostomy
- Vasoepididymostomy • History • Vasectomy
- Microsurgery

With the application of vasectomy for eugenic, punitive, and therapeutic purposes gaining momentum in the early part of the twentieth century,[1] a new surgical procedure, the vasectomy reversal, was born. The dawn of the vasectomy procedure was marred by dubious scientific and at times overtly sinister elements. Although the history of vasectomy is discussed in another article in this issue, a brief discussion of the development of the vasectomy procedure is pertinent to this discussion of vasectomy reversal. Vasectomies in the early 1900s were not as they are today, a safe and effective method of voluntary contraception; they often were performed for medically questionable reasons, such as severe prostatic hypertrophy[2] and physical and mental revitalization through the Steinach rejuvenation procedure,[3] and for political motives, such as eugenics[4] and punitive sterilization of criminals.[1,5] The medical principle of *primum non nocere* was not always followed in the early years of this procedure. The Nazi mass sterilization effort during World War II was merely the culmination of decades of medical demagoguery and misapplication of the vasectomy procedure.

Vincent J. O'Conor, Chicago urologist and former chairman of the Department of Urology at Northwestern University Medical School, posited that these political underpinnings were the spurs that promoted considerable interest in the vasectomy reversal procedure by the medical and nonmedical communities, including members of religious groups.[6] As of 1948, however, O'Conor observed that most people assumed that reversal surgery was hardly worth considering, given the technical challenges and low success rates.[6] Because urologic surgeons still approached this relatively untested reversal procedure with trepidation and because of the political, religious, and personal implications of vasectomy surgery, men undergoing vasectomy and its reversal often did so under a cloak of secrecy.[6] Furthermore, the legality of this procedure was in question in most states, and urologists performing the surgery were at risk for legal challenges and malpractice suits.[6] In his brief article, O'Conor provides a fascinating glimpse into the practice of male reproductive medicine in post–World War II society.

"FOUNDING FATHER OF MODERN CLINICAL ANDROLOGY"

The birth of the reversal procedure goes back even further than O'Conor's era. A history of surgical reversal rightfully begins with the work of Edward Martin, Chief Surgeon at the University of Pennsylvania during the early years of the past century, although technically he performed vasoepididymostomies in men who had obstruction secondary to epididymitis, not vasectomy (**Fig. 1**). In 1902, Martin reported the first

Funding source for this article was The Frederick J. and Theresa Dow Wallace Fund of the New York Community Trust.

a Department of Urology, Cornell Institute for Reproductive Medicine, New York-Presbyterian Hospital/Weill Cornell Medical Center, Weill Cornell Medical College, Box 580, 525 East 68th Street, New York, NY 10065, USA
b Male Reproductive Medicine and Surgery, Cornell Institute for Reproductive Medicine, New York-Presbyterian Hospital/Weill Cornell Medical Center, Weill Cornell Medical College, 525 East 68th Street, Box 580, New York, NY 10065, USA
c The Population Council, Center for Biomedical Research, New York, NY 10065, USA
* Corresponding author. Cornell Institute for Reproductive Medicine, New York-Presbyterian Hospital/Weill Cornell Medical Center, Weill Cornell Medical College, 525 East 68th Street, Box 580, New York, NY 10065.
E-mail address: mgoldst@med.cornell.edu (M. Goldstein).

Urol Clin N Am 36 (2009) 359–373
doi:10.1016/j.ucl.2009.05.001

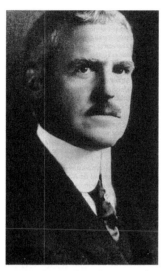

Fig. 1. A portrait of Dr. Edward Martin. (*From* Jequier AM. Edward Martin [1859–1938]. The founding father of modern clinical andrology. Int J Androl 1991;14:1, [reprinted from the Public Ledger, 1914].)

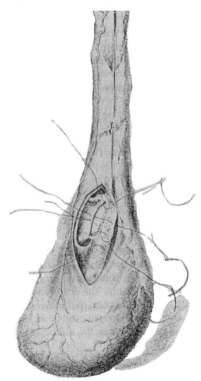

Fig. 2. A Martin's vasoepididymostomy surgery. (*From* Jequier AM. Edward Martin [1859–1938]. The founding father of modern clinical andrology. Int J Androl 1991;14:1.)

documented vasoepididymostomy in his study of 192 sterile couples and examination of sperm morphology.[7,8] He initially performed the procedure on three dogs before operating on a man who had obstructive azoospermia.[7] The following year, Martin reported his case of unilateral side-to-side vasoepididymostomy in a man who had a history of epididymitis and gonococcal urethritis, which resulted in sperm in the ejaculate and the birth of a full-term infant.[7,9] After incising the epididymis at a location yielding exudation of milky fluid, Martin constructed the vasal-epididymal fistula using four fine silver wire sutures brought from the outer surface of the vas deferens into the lumen and then through the cut surface of the epididymis and its tunic (**Fig. 2**).[7–9] In 1909, Martin published his series of 15 azoospermic men who had obstructive lesions, 11 who had epididymal and 4 who had vasal obstruction.[7,10] Possible origins of azoospermia in these men included orchitis (nonobstructive azoospermia), congenital absence of the vasa deferentia, secondary vasal atrophy, long vasal stricture, and distal vasa or ejaculatory duct obstruction.[7] Martin performed vasoepididymostomies in the 11 men who had epididymal obstruction using the same technique described in his previous publication, with patency and pregnancy rates of 64% and 27%, respectively.[7] Not only did Martin demonstrate the effectiveness of the reconstructive procedure for obstructive azoospermia but also he observed that azoospermia can be obstructive and nonobstructive.[7] Martin's clinical acumen was remarkable, and his observations

seem to fit current standards of reproductive medicine rather than those of 1909. He even checked vasal patency during the vasoepididymostomy procedure, foretelling today's use of vasography. The significance of his contributions to the field of male infertility inspired Jequier to entitle Martin the "founding father of modern clinical andrology" in her profile piece.[7]

Francis Hagner of Washington, DC, was an early proponent of Martin's surgery. In 1907, Hagner reported at the twenty-first annual meeting of the American Association of Genito-Urinary Surgeons two cases of successful anastomosis between the vas deferens and the globus major; one surgery had been performed by Martin and the other by Hagner.[11] The surgery was performed with fine silver wire and curved intestinal needles, and the vas deferens was anastomosed to the epididymis after observation of white fluid exudation from a small wedge-shaped incision in the globus major. Sperm was detected in the ejaculate at 1 month. Hagner's continued success with the vasoepididymal anastomosis helped popularize the procedure.[12] In 1936 he reported patency and pregnancy rates of 64% and 48%, respectively, in 33 patients undergoing vasoepididymostomy.[13]

Hagner's technique was modified and used by Hanley in Great Britain and Bayle in France.[12,14,15]

CAPACITY FOR REGENERATION

H. C. Rolnick was another Chicago urologist at Northwestern University Medical School who contributed to the development of vasectomy and reconstructive surgery. In 1924, he published his series of 48 vasal surgeries in 25 dogs, in which he ligated, incised, or resected the vasa to determine their regenerative capacity.[16] In the five dogs in which both vasa were ligated with catgut suture, all vasa were patent when checked after 21 to 38 days. In one of the dogs, the left vas deferens was sutured to the skin and a horsehair was left in the lumen, but this did not prevent patency. When Rolnick made multiple longitudinal and oblique incisions of the vasa, three of five were patent. Multiple transverse incisions of the vas always resulted in occlusion of the lumen. When six vasa were divided and separated from the sheath, however, no patency was observed. In contrast, six of seven vasa achieved patency when divided without disturbing the sheath or deferential vessels. Foreign body or suture in the lumen did not cause occlusion. In several dogs, Rolnick performed reversal surgery of the divided vasa and achieved patency in five of 13 anastomoses. From these results, he concluded that the vas deferens had the ability to resist trauma and restore its luminal patency and the intact vasal sheath and deferential vessels play an important role in the restoration of vasal integrity after injury.

VASOVASOSTOMY

In 1919, Quinby reported the first successful vasovasostomy in a man who had undergone bilateral vas resection in 1911.[6] He created the anastomosis over a strand of silkworm gut, which was removed after 10 days.[17] Quinby's assistant for this historic procedure was none other than O'Conor. O'Conor subsequently used Quinby's technique in 14 vasectomized patients, resulting in a patency rate of 64%.[6] In the same article published in 1948, O'Conor reported the results of his survey of 1240 urologists on the topic of vasectomy reversals. Seven hundred fifty urologists completed the questionnaire, and only 135 had any experience with the procedure. Of the 420 reported operations, patency rate was 38%, although the rate of spontaneous recanalization of the vasa was not determined.[6] Several such surveys have been conducted in the ensuing decades, and this report provides the first snapshot of clinical practice patterns for vasectomy reversal surgery.

By the 1970s, many reports on macrosurgical techniques for vasovasostomy began appearing in the literature. Hulka and Davis reviewed vasovasostomy series from the United States, India, and Denmark and compiled 705 cases. They found a patency rate of 60% and a pregnancy rate of 44% in series reporting pregnancies.[18] The investigators discussed pertinent anatomic considerations, such as the average luminal diameter of the vas deferens (0.55 mm) having significant variation and pondered whether or not ligation of the sympathetic nerve fibers of the inferior spermatic nerve during vasectomy resulted in permanent impairment of sperm transport through the vas deferens.[18] They also reviewed methods for reversible vasocclusion, including use of prosthetic plugs with injections of Silastic and other nonreactive synthetic materials, an intra vas device similar in theory to the intrauterine device, and the vas clip and vas valve.[18] Even within the confines of this scientific review article, hints of the broader political and social context of vasectomy and vasectomy reversal during the 1970s surfaced, with references to the zero population growth movement and allusions to the second wave of the feminist movement.[18] Interest in vasectomy flourished during this time because of increased interest in family planning by men and the emancipation of women.[18] With the increasing popularity of vasectomy, the relevance of vasectomy reversals inevitably followed.

In 1973, Getzoff published another questionnaire study of 150 urologists, examining their views and management of reversal surgery.[19] On the topic of vasoepididymostomy, 13.3% had never performed this procedure, 28% had had no success, 20.7% rare (1%) success, 21.3% occasional (5%) success, 14% moderate (20%) success, and 2.7% moderately encouraging success (50% to 70% reported in the literature). When indications for a vasoepididymostomy were present, 9.3% urologists encouraged the operation, 27.3% discouraged it, and 63.3% had discussions with the patients about the procedure and prognosis. The same questions were asked regarding vasovasostomy, and 6% had never performed this procedure, 8% had had no success, 11.3% rare (1%) success, 20% occasional (5%) success, 38.7% moderate (20%) success, and 16% encouraging success (50% to 70% reported in the literature). When a patient presented for a potential vasovasostomy, 8.7% urologists encouraged the operation, 5.3% discouraged it, and 86% had discussions about the procedure and prognosis. Sixty-two percent believed a second procedure should not be attempted if the initial reversal surgery failed. Regarding surgical technique, no splint was used in 9.9% of cases, silver wire in 51.1%, nylon suture in 33.8%, Silastic tubing in 9.5%, steel wire in 3.2%, silk suture in 0.8%, and other splints in 1.6%. Compared with the results from O'Conor's survey in 1948, there was a dramatic increase in the proportion of urologists who had at least some experience with reversal surgery. Perhaps more telling is the stark contrast between the published success rates in the literature (50% to 70%) and the low success rates in actual clinical practice.

ETIOLOGIES OF VASECTOMY REVERSAL FAILURE

Since the early studies of Rolnick, several groups have studied the causes of reversal surgery failures. Failures can be functional or anatomic.

Functional Failure: Agglutinating Antibodies

Sullivan and Howe tested the serum of 45 men who had sperm in their ejaculate after reversal surgery and found agglutinating antibodies in 48% of those whose partners became pregnant and in 94% of those whose partners did not ($P < .01$).[20] The investigators did not believe, however, autoagglutination to be the mechanism for immunologic infertility in functional reversal failures because almost half of fertile men had the antibodies, autoagglutination of sperm was not seen in any of the study patients, and previous evidence had demonstrated in a rabbit model that immunologically induced sperm agglutination is neither necessary nor sufficient for sperm deactivation.[20] In contrast, Requeda and colleagues[21] concluded that sperm antibodies are an important cause of infertility in men who have undergone reversal surgery. In their study, six of eight fertile reversal patients had low titers of serum agglutinins, normal fertilizing capacity of their sperm, and no immobilizing antibodies, whereas six of seven infertile reversal patients had elevated serum agglutinins and four had agglutinating antibodies in seminal plasma and serum immobilizing antibodies.[21]

Anatomic Failure: Sperm Granuloma

The effect of sperm granulomas on reversal surgery outcomes also has been evaluated. Working with a dog model, Schmidt determined that causes of vasovasostomy failure included sperm granuloma formation resulting from anastomotic leakage of sperm secondary to inadequate approximation of the vasal ends, puncture of the vasal lumen, misalignment of the anastomosis, and infection.[22] Hagan and Coffey performed 119 vasovasostomies on 95 rats and found that sperm granulomas were present in 99% of the 49 failed anastomoses.[23] They also performed vasal anastomoses in immature animals or in adult animals with suppression of spermatogenesis with testosterone and achieved 95% patency without granulomas.[23] Alexander and Schmidt reported that more men who had sperm granulomas had sperm-immobilizing antibodies.[24]

A healthy, patent epididymis is the cornerstone of successful vasectomy reversal surgery. Silber microsurgically explored the epididymis of 28 men undergoing vasectomy reversal who were found to have no sperm in the vasal fluid of the testicular side of the vas deferens.[25] Sperm was found in 33 of 39 epididymides and histologic evaluation distal to the area with sperm revealed extensive interstitial sperm granulomas resulting from epididymal duct rupture.[25] He concluded that persistent azoospermia after vasovasostomy resulted from secondary epididymal obstruction due to epididymal duct rupture from increased pressure after vasectomy.[25]

Functional and technical problems do not account for all reversal failures. Continued infertility after surgery may be unrelated to surgical technique. For example, the epididymis also is important because of its role in sperm maturation. Schoysman and Bedford reported a greater chance of pregnancy after vasoepididymostomy with anastomosis to the corpus instead of the caput, with motility the only sperm characteristic affected.[26] In most men whose anastomosis was located 8 mm or less from the proximal border of the caput, sperm were immotile.[26] In contrast, 20% to 90% of sperm were progressively motile in cases where the anastomosis were greater than 10 mm from the caput border.[26]

MACROSURGICAL TECHNIQUE

A wide range of macrosurgical techniques for vasovasostomy has been reported. The main variation in technique seems to be the use or omission of loupe magnification and stenting. Stenting is the use of a suture, tube, or other foreign body to help keep the lumen of the vas deferens open after a reversal procedure. Stents usually but not always are removed during the postoperative period.

Amelar and Dubin favored a nonstented technique with 4× loupe magnification using eight 6-0 Prolene sutures.[27] Once the vas is exposed and the scarred ends are excised, the distal vas is cannulated with a blunt needle and tested for patency by injecting hydrogen peroxide dyed with methylene blue.[27] Fluid from the proximal vas is examined with microscopy for the presence of sperm.[27] These investigators used a stent to assist during the anastomosis but did not leave the stent in place to aid in healing. A 2-0 nylon suture is used as a stent during the creation of the anastomosis with the eight 6-0 Prolene sutures and is always removed before closure.[27] This procedure is similar to the Schmidt operation,[28] from which many of the derivative techniques have been adapted.

In contrast, Dorsey described a stented technique without magnification.[29] He used a blunt 20-gauge needle with obturator to pierce the wall of the proximal vas, 1 centimeter from the site of anastomosis and the fascia, dartos, and scrotal skin. A zero monofilament dermalon suture is fed through the needle and the other end of the suture is advanced 12 to 14 cm into the distal vas segment. The anastomosis is formed over the stenting suture with four or five 6-0 Ethiflex sutures. The dartos layer is closed with a running 3-0 chromic suture. The stenting suture is exteriorized through the scrotal skin and is threaded through two lead shots, and the shots are crimped to keep the suture in place. The stenting suture is removed in 12 to 14 days, based on Schmidt's finding that 7 to 10 days are required for epithelialization of the anastomosis.[30] Dorsey reported successful reversal of vasectomy in 88% of 129 patients undergoing this procedure, including one patient who was 19 years post vasectomy.[29]

Fitzpatrick reported the flap technique in 1978, in which both vasal ends are bivalved to create flaps.[31] These flaps permanently widen the opening into each vasal lumen, resulting in a ballooning of the lumen at the site of anastomosis. In his preliminary study of 14 men, all had sperm in their ejaculate by postoperative week 6, and a 50% pregnancy rate was achieved by 3 months.[31] Singh and Sharma used the Fitzpatrick flap operation with 2.5× magnification in 40 men and achieved patency and pregnancy rates of 79% and 34%, respectively.[32] They proposed this spatulation technique as an alternative to the microsurgical approach for those without microsurgical training.

TO STENT OR NOT TO STENT

Although "stent" and "splint" have been used interchangeably in the literature to describe the use of a foreign material to encourage patency of the vasal lumen during the time of epithelialization of the anastomosis, Montie and colleagues[33] pointed out that a splint refers to something placed outside a structure to stabilize it whereas a stent is a compound for holding some form of graft in place. Stent, therefore, is the more accurate descriptor in this context. The use of exteriorized stents has several potential disadvantages, including infection and sperm leakage.[33] Stents can provide a portal of entry for bacteria and serve as a foreign body to perpetuate the infection. Montie and colleagues[33] tested in a canine model the feasibility of a completely intravasal stent using absorbable suture that does not require postoperative removal. Nineteen dogs underwent vasovasostomies with and without intravasal stents. The group without intravasal stents had a patency rate of 50% compared to 60% patency in the Dexon intravasal stent group and 70% patency in the chromic intravasal stent group.[33] Rowland and colleagues[34] confirmed these findings in 35 patients, with 86% patency using 3-0 plain catgut internal stents compared to 67% patency with externalized silkworm gut stents. The investigators pointed out, however, that patency rates varied widely by series: 60% to 67% for externalized gut stents,[6,34,35] 83% to 95% for externalized nylon stents,[36-38] 78% for intraoperative stainless steel stents,[39] 92% for Silastic tube stents,[40] and 100% for no stenting.[41]

Using O'Conor's 1948 questionnaire study as a model, Derrick and colleagues[42] sent a survey to every member of the American Urological Association (2775 questionnaires). Of the 1363 replies, 542 urologists (40%) had performed at least one reversal procedure. The overall patency and pregnancy rates were 38% and 19.5%, respectively.[42] This survey addressed the impact of stents on reconstructive success. The pregnancy rate for nonstented reversals was 10.9% compared to 19.9% to 26% for stented procedures (depending on the stent used).[42]

The use of stents was the preferred method between 1940 and 1975.[43,44] The disadvantages of stents were reported, including Fernandes and colleagues' demonstration in dogs that obstruction often occurred at the site of exit of the stent through the vas deferens instead of at the anastomosis.[45,46] As surgical technique improved with the widespread availability of microsurgery, stents gradually disappeared from reversal surgery.

MICROSURGICAL TECHNIQUE

Owen[47] and Silber,[48,49] working independently, are credited with the development of the microsurgical vasovasostomy technique for clinical use. The use of the microscope for the anastomosis of the vas deferens in animals had been previously evaluated by several groups.[46,50,51] The earliest reference to microsurgical vasovasostomy in humans was by Silber in 1975.[52] Most of the initial animal studies involved a one-layer anastomosis, but Silber determined that in humans a two-layer is preferable largely because of the discrepant luminal diameters due to dilatation of the proximal vas segment.[53] Silber performed the anastomosis under 16× to 25× magnification using single-armed 9-0 nylon sutures (**Fig. 3**). He dilated the abdominal portion of the vas deferens with the insertion of jeweler's forceps. The mucosal sutures included the elastic layer subjacent to the mucosa. After placement and tying of the three anterior sutures, the clamp is flipped to visualize the posterior wall of the anastomosis. He advocated careful inspection for gaps, tears, or inaccuracy of the lineup after placement of the six or seven mucosal sutures. The outer muscularis layer is then sutured separately. The two-layer technique allows for superior mucosal approximation and leakproof closure.[53] Silber and colleagues[41] performed histologic and electron microscopic studies and found that stricture was a common cause of failure with conventional or nonmicroscopic vasovasostomies and that obstruction of the vas deferens inhibited spermatogenesis. Further refinements to this microsurgical technique have been made over the years, including Goldstein's introduction of the microspike approximator clamp (**Fig. 4**)[54] and use of microdots for precision suture placement.[55] By providing a blueprint for the anastomosis, the dots minimize gaps and distortions of

the anastomosis even with discrepant sizes of the cut vasal ends (**Fig. 5**).

In 2004, Silber and Grotjan summarized their experience with 4010 cases of microscopic vasectomy reversal.[56] Of 1357 patients undergoing microsurgical vasovasostomy, patency was achieved in 94.4%. Of 1008 patients undergoing unilateral vasoepididymostomy (with contralateral vasovasostomy) and 1013 patients undergoing bilateral vasoepididymostomy, patency rates were 93.7% and 78.7%, respectively.

In 1980, Lee and McLoughlin reported their comparison of macroscopic and microscopic vasovasostomy techniques.[57] The macroscopic anastomoses were performed with a nonabsorbable monofilament internal stent, which was removed 7 to 14 days postoperatively and four to six absorbable sutures sized 4-0 to 6-0. The microsurgical anastomoses were performed in two layers using 8-0 to 10-0 synthetic suture. For the 61 patients undergoing the single-layer macroscopic procedure, patency and pregnancy rates were 90% and 46%, respectively. For the 26 patients undergoing the two-layer microscopic procedure, the rates were 96% and 54%, respectively. The investigators reported 100% patency and an 88% pregnancy rate in patients undergoing reversal surgery less than 2 years after the initial vasectomy and postulated importance of the 2-year period. Similarly, Silber had previously

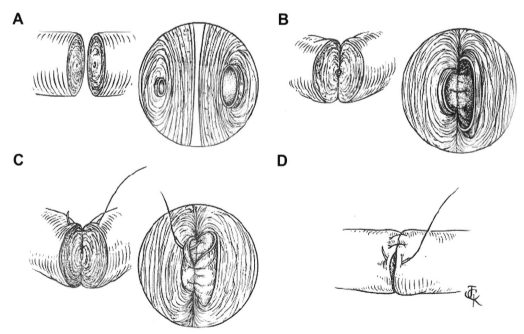

Fig. 3. The steps in Silber's microscopic technique of vasovasostomy. (*A*) The lumen is inspected for patency. (*B, C*) Mucosal anastomosis. (*D*) Separate anastomosis of muscularis. (*From* Silber SJ. Microscopic technique for reversal of vasectomy. Surg Gynecol Obstet 1967;143:631, copyright Elsevier; with permission.)

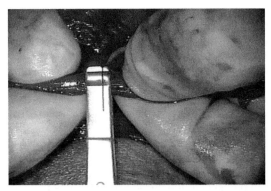

Fig. 4. The slotted nerve holding clamp for making a perfect 90° transection of the vas deferens. (*Courtesy of* Marc Goldstein, MD, New York, NY.)

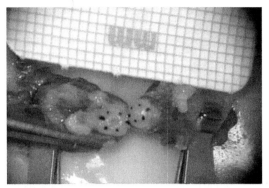

Fig. 5. A photograph of the microdot technique of precision suture placement, demonstrating the large lumen of the testicular vas and the small lumen of the abdominal vas. (*Courtesy of* Marc Goldstein, MD, New York, NY.)

reported in 1977 the importance of duration of obstruction, with improved patency rates in those undergoing reversal surgery less than 10 years from the original vasectomy.[48] Although opinion of the precise time interval between initial vasectomy and subsequent reversal has since changed, Lee and McLoughlin recognized the significance of the time interval to reversal outcomes. In 2004, Boorjian and colleagues[58] reassessed obstructive intervals and determined that the pregnancy rate was significantly lower in those whose vasectomy had been performed more than 15 years before reversal surgery. Pregnancy rates were 89%, 82%, and 86% for obstructive intervals of 0 to 5, 5 to 10 and 10 to 15 years, respectively, compared to 44% for obstructive intervals greater than 15 years. Furthermore, Fuchs and Burt reported that spousal age is an important predictive factor after vasectomy reversal when surgery is performed 15 years or more after vasectomy.[59]

The impact of the obstructive interval has been addressed by another important series published by the Vasovasostomy Study Group in 1991.[60] The Vasovasostomy Study Group was a consortium of five institutions that pooled data for a 9-year period for a total of 1469 microsurgical vasectomy reversal procedures. Of the 1012 men who underwent reversal surgery for the first time and presented for postoperative semen analysis, 865 (86%) achieved patency. Four hundred twenty-one (52%) of 810 couples achieved pregnancy. The patency and pregnancy rates declined as the interval between the vasectomy and the reversal surgery increased: 97% and 76%, respectively, for interval less than 3 years, compared to 71% and 30%, respectively, for intervals greater than 15 years.

In 2004, Crain and colleagues[61] published another questionnaire study on the practice patterns of vasectomy reversal surgery among

practicing urologists and highlighted the significance of obstructive intervals. They received 622 completed questionnaires from 1508 mailed. Of the 59% who performed vasectomy reversals, 8% were fellowship trained in infertility, 23% were affiliated with residency training, and 69% practiced in a community setting, with fellowship-trained urologists performing more reversal procedures per year than the others.[61] Fellowship-trained urologists also were more likely to perform surgery on patients greater than 15 years since vasectomy.[61] Compared with the other two groups, they also were more likely to use the operating microscope (93% versus 65% and 56%) and examine the vasal fluid (83% versus 75% and 67%) and to use finer suture material.[61]

ONE LAYER OR TWO?

Microsurgical vasovasostomy began as a double-layer technique and was quickly established as the gold standard. As with all surgical procedures, however, modifications were promoted as improvements on the original. Inevitably, several groups promoted the single-layer technique as a simpler alternative. Schroeder-Printzen and colleagues[62] reviewed the outcomes for several series of double-layer and single-layer reversal surgeries. Patency and pregnancy rates (mean ±SD) in 12 series comprising 2183 cases of double-layer vasovasostomies were 87% ± 13 and 52% ± 17, respectively.[55,62–73] In four series of single-layer vasovasostomies with 185 cases, patency and pregnancy rates (mean ±SD) were 90% ± 8 and 53% ± 10, respectively.[62,74–76] They also reviewed five series in which the two techniques were compared. Patency and pregnancy rates (mean ±SD) for 724 single-layer cases were 89% ± 8 and 56% ± 12, respectively, and 91% ± 5 and 57% ± 12, respectively, for 902 double-layer cases.[60,62,77–80] It is difficult to draw conclusions from these data, as the constituent studies had heterogeneous methodology, patient populations, and surgeon experience. Outcomes reported by the Vasovasostomy Study Group for double-layer and modified single-layer anastomoses were statistically the same.[60]

VASOGRAPHY

Vasography had been in use for many years, as far back as 1909 by Martin (discussed previously). Although Martin used vasography to confirm patency of the distal vas deferens before performing an anastomosis of the vas deferens to the epididymis in a similar fashion to vasograms of today, vasography also has been used to test the anastomosis, more in line with the use of vasograms in a laboratory setting or microsurgical training.

In 1982, Hartig and Meyer assessed the safety of intraoperative vasography at the time of vasovasostomy.[81] They evaluated the use of vasography in 11 cases when dissatisfaction with the appearance of one of their anastomosis prompted them to perform an intraoperative vasogram. They used the vasogram technique described by Paulson and coworkers,[82] which involved gentle injection of 6 mL of contrast material into the vas deferens. A radiograph was obtained simultaneously with the injection and the film was evaluated for demonstration of contrast material across the anastomosis. No complications were observed, and all patients had return of sperm in their ejaculates. This contrasted with the experience of Jenkins and Blacklock, who performed intraoperative vasography in one patient who developed a mild postoperative epididymitis.[83]

VASOEPIDIDYMOSTOMY

Vasoepididymostomy techniques can be broadly categorized as "fistula formation" based on Martin's original technique or "tubule-to-tubule" as described by Silber.[84] As Thomas pointed out, although Silber generally is credited for the single tubule-to-tubule anastomosis, Lespinasse had a similar idea 60 years earlier, wherein a 5-0 silk suture was passed through a single epididymal loop and the mucosal surface of the vasal lumen.[84,85]

In 1978, Silber described his technique involving the direct end-to-end anastomosis of the inner lumen of the vas deferens to one epididymal tubule.[86] The epididymis is inspected under 10× to 16× magnification, allowing for identification of tubules dilated to 0.1 to 0.2 mm in diameter secondary to obstruction.[86] Approximately 1 cm of the epididymis is dissected from the testis, and the vas deferens is prepared in the same fashion as for a vasovasostomy. Under 16× to 25× magnification, the epididymis is transected completely at the lowest point, and, although multiple epididymal tubules are cut, the appropriate tubule is selected by efflux of sperm fluid with microscopy to check for presence of sperm.[86] If no efflux of sperm fluid is encountered, another transection of the epididymis is made 0.5 cm proximal to the previous cut.[86] So by trial and error, the epididymis is sequentially sampled from the distal portion to the proximal portion. The anastomosis is created using interrupted 9-0 or 10-0 nylon sutures, with the first two sutures placed posteriorly from the outside in on the epididymal tubule.[86] These sutures then are placed from inside the mucosa of the vas deferens to the outside and tied. The two anterior sutures are placed in a similar manner.[86] The muscularis of the vas deferens is approximated to the epididymal tunic using 10 to 12 9-0 nylon sutures to provide stability for the delicate mucosal anastomosis.[86] In his preliminary group of 14 patients, 12 (86%) had sperm counts of greater than 20 million per mL.[86] In a follow-up study, Silber observed that patients who had undergone microsurgical vasoepididymostomy of the proximal (head) region of the epididymis had poor sperm motility, which improved within 1.5 to 2 years.[87]

Many variations of this end-to-end anastomosis have been developed, but the end-to-end approach gradually fell out favor with the advancement of end-to-side techniques, in which a single epididymal loop is isolated and the anterior wall of the loop is unroofed for the anastomosis to the vas deferens. Resection of the epididymis for end-to-end anastomosis can result in bleeding and difficulty identifying a patent tubule. Wagenknecht was one of the early advocates of the end-to-side technique.[88] In 1998, Berger published his triangulation end-to-side technique, which involves placement of three double-armed 10-0 nylon sutures into the epididymis so that each suture forms one side of a triangle.[89] An opening is made in the epididymal tubule and the sutures are brought inside-out, invaginating the tubule into the vasal lumen.[89] Ninety-two percent patency was achieved in 12 men with this technique.[89] In 2003, Chan and colleagues[90] introduced the two-suture longitudinal technique, in which two double-armed 10-0 nylon sutures are placed longitudinally along the anterior surface of a single epididymal tubule. The needles are pulled through only after the tubular opening is made. The sutures are placed into the vas deferens from inside out at four points and, when the sutures are tied, the epididymal tubule intussuscepts into the vasal lumen. Using a rat model, the group reported comparable outcomes for this technique compared with other two or three suture intussusception vasoepididymostomy techniques, with the advantage of a larger opening in the epididymal tubule and shorter operative time.[90]

REVERSAL SURGERY IN THE AGE OF ASSISTED REPRODUCTION

Despite progress over the years with vasectomy reversal, the introduction of intracytoplasmic sperm injection (ICSI) led many to wonder if technically challenging microsurgical vasectomy reversals were worth the trouble. There are several important advantages to reversal surgery, including treatment of an affected man instead of his healthy partner, natural conception through sexual intercourse, and the ability to father more than one child after one procedure. If an experienced microsurgeon is available, the biggest downside to reversal surgery is the length of time for return of sperm to the ejaculate, which can take 6 months to 2 years or longer.[68] In the fast-paced modern era, time is of the essence, and many fertility clinics bypass consideration of reversal surgery. Comparisons of reversal surgery to ICSI have been studied, however, and the results usually favor reversal surgery. Pavlovich and Schlegel conducted a cost-effectiveness analysis of vasectomy reversal and ICSI and determined that cost per delivery with an initial approach of vasectomy reversal was $25,475 (95% CI, $19,609 to $31,339) with a delivery rate of 47% compared with cost per delivery after sperm retrieval and ICSI of $72,521 (95% CI, $63,357 to $81,685) with a delivery rate after one cycle of sperm retrieval of 33%.[91] Microsurgical reversal surgery provided the most cost-effective treatment for postvasectomy infertility and the highest chance of resulting in delivery of a child for a single intervention. Kolettis and Thomas concurred that vasoepididymostomy is more successful and cost-effective than ICSI with retrieved sperm.[92]

THE FUTURE?

Surgical procedures are forever evolving, whether or not it is a simplification of mechanics or the application of new technology, surgeons always are looking for ways to streamline an operation and to nudge up success rates while reducing complications. Because suturing of the anastomosis is the most technically challenging step in the vasectomy reversal procedure, a wide variety of sutureless anastomotic techniques has been evaluated, including laser welding,[93,94] microclip,[95] fibrin glue,[96,97] and other biomaterials as surgical sealants.[98] Sutureless techniques are still in the experimental stage with animal studies, and some time may pass before a suitable biomaterial is available for clinical use.

Urology has entered the robotic age. The da Vinci robotic system has captured the imagination of the public, enraptured by the space age concept of having a cancerous organ removed by a hulking but benevolent robot under the remote control of a genius scientist cum surgeon. Will reversal surgery follow urologic oncology down the technology path? Perhaps. Several groups have considered this possibility, including Schiff and colleagues,[99] who randomized 24 rats to undergo microsurgical multilayer vasovasostomy, longitudinal vasoepididymostomy or robotic vasovasostomy, and vasoepididymostomy. To perform the robotic procedure, the anastomosis was set up using a conventional operating microscope and transferred to the robotic field to undergo the anastomosis. Patency rates were 100% for the robotic approach and 90% for the microsurgical approach (no statistical difference). Robotic vasovasostomy was significantly faster than conventional microsurgical technique, 68.5 versus 102.5 minutes (P = .002). The investigators concluded that the robotic approach improved stability and motion reduction and provided the potential for microsurgeons to perform reversal surgery in patients at remote locations lacking access to experienced microsurgeons. Advances in medical technology always are tempered, however, by cost considerations. The cost-effectiveness of the application of robotic technology to infertility surgery remains to be determined.

SUMMARY

Vasectomy reversal has come a long way since Martin performed the first anastomosis of the vas deferens and epididymis. Although its history is not as politically charged as that of vasectomy, the progress of reversal surgery has had its share of ups and downs, brilliant discoveries, and discouraging missteps (see Appendix). In the early part of the twentieth century, vasovasostomy and vasoepididymostomy were esoteric procedures, but by the 1970s, a majority of urologists had at least some experience with reversal surgery, although not as successfully as reported in the literature. With the advent of the microsurgical technique, reversal surgery increasingly has become once more a specialist's undertaking. The history of vasectomy reversal is an excellent case study in the evolution of surgery, rich with leaders, innovators, and pioneers.

ACKNOWLEDGMENTS

We thank Vanessa Lynne Dudley for creating the timeline layout in the Appendix.

APPENDIX: TIMELINE OF THE HISTORY OF REVERSAL SURGERY

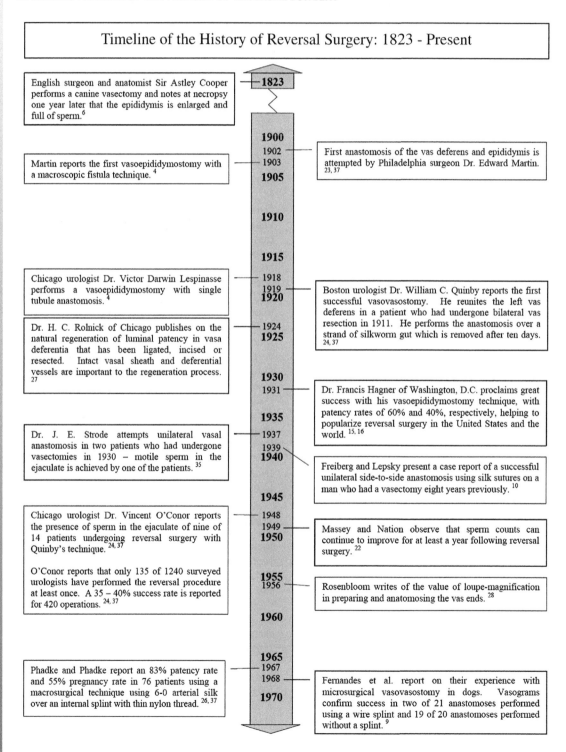

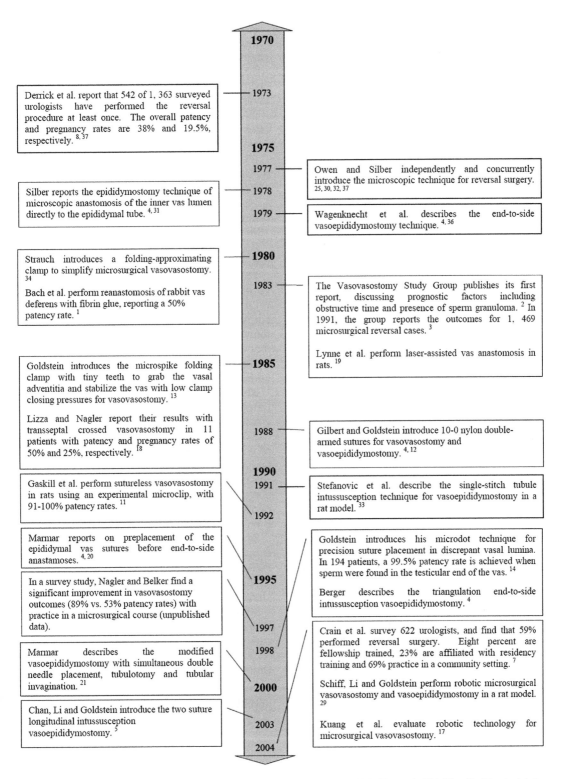

1970

Derrick et al. report that 542 of 1, 363 surveyed urologists have performed the reversal procedure at least once. The overall patency and pregnancy rates are 38% and 19.5%, respectively. [8, 37]

1973

1975

1977 — Owen and Silber independently and concurrently introduce the microscopic technique for reversal surgery. [25, 30, 32, 37]

1978 — Silber reports the epididymostomy technique of microscopic anastomosis of the inner vas lumen directly to the epididymal tube. [4, 31]

1979 — Wagenknecht et al. describes the end-to-side vasoepididymostomy technique. [4, 36]

1980 — Strauch introduces a folding-approximating clamp to simplify microsurgical vasovasostomy. [34]

Bach et al. perform reanastomosis of rabbit vas deferens with fibrin glue, reporting a 50% patency rate. [1]

1983 — The Vasovasostomy Study Group publishes its first report, discussing prognostic factors including obstructive time and presence of sperm granuloma. [2] In 1991, the group reports the outcomes for 1, 469 microsurgical reversal cases. [3]

Lynne et al. perform laser-assisted vas anastomosis in rats. [19]

1985 — Goldstein introduces the microspike folding clamp with tiny teeth to grab the vasal adventitia and stabilize the vas with low clamp closing pressures for vasovasostomy. [13]

Lizza and Nagler report their results with transseptal crossed vasovasostomy in 11 patients with patency and pregnancy rates of 50% and 25%, respectively. [18]

1988 — Gilbert and Goldstein introduce 10-0 nylon double-armed sutures for vasovasostomy and vasoepididymostomy. [4, 12]

1990

1991 — Stefanovic et al. describe the single-stitch tubule intussusception technique for vasoepididymostomy in a rat model. [33]

Gaskill et al. perform sutureless vasovasostomy in rats using an experimental microclip, with 91-100% patency rates. [11]

1992

Marmar reports on preplacement of the epididymal vas sutures before end-to-side anastamoses. [4, 20]

Goldstein introduces his microdot technique for precision suture placement in discrepant vasal lumina. In 194 patients, a 99.5% patency rate is achieved when sperm were found in the testicular end of the vas. [14]

In a survey study, Nagler and Belker find a significant improvement in vasovasostomy outcomes (89% vs. 53% patency rates) with practice in a microsurgical course (unpublished data).

1995 — Berger describes the triangulation end-to-side intussusception vasoepididymostomy. [4]

1997

1998 — Crain et al. survey 622 urologists, and find that 59% performed reversal surgery. Eight percent are fellowship trained, 23% are affiliated with residency training and 69% practice in a community setting. [7]

Marmar describes the modified vasoepididymostomy with simultaneous double needle placement, tubulotomy and tubular invagination. [21]

2000 — Schiff, Li and Goldstein perform robotic microsurgical vasovasostomy and vasoepididymostomy in a rat model. [29]

Chan, Li and Goldstein introduce the two suture longitudinal intussusception vasoepididymostomy. [5]

2003 — Kuang et al. evaluate robotic technology for microsurgical vasovasostomy. [17]

2004

APPENDIX: REFERENCES

1. Bach D, Distelmaier W, Weissbach L. Animal experiments on reanastomosis of the vas deferens using fibrin glue. Urol Res 1980;8:29–36.

2. Belker AM, Konnak JW, Sharlip ID, et al. Intraoperative observations during vasovasostomy in 334 patients. J Urol 1983;129:524–7.

3. Belker AM, Thomas Jr. AJ, Fuchs EF, et al. Results of 1,469 microsurgical vasectomy

reversals by the Vasovasostomy Study Group. J Urol 1991;145:505–11.

4. Berger RE. Triangulation end-to-side vasoepididymostomy. J Urol 1998;159:1951–3.

5. Chan PT, Li PS, Goldstein M. Microsurgical vasoepididymostomy: a prospective randomized study of 3 intussusception techniques in rats. J Urol 2003;169:1924–9.

6. Cos LR, Valvo JR, Davis RS, et al. Vasovasostomy: current state of the art. Urology 1983;22:567–75.

7. Crain DS, Roberts JL, Amling CL. Practice patterns in vasectomy reversal surgery: results of a questionnaire study among practicing urologists. J Urol 2004;171:311–5.

8. Derrick FC Jr. Yarbrough W, D'Agostino J. Vasovasostomy: results of questionnaire of members of the American Urological Association. J Urol 1973;110:556–7.

9. Fernandes M, Shah KN, Draper JW. Vasovasostomy: improved microsurgical technique. J Urol 1968;100:763–6.

10. Freiberg HB, Lepsky HO. Restoration of the continuity of the vas deferens eight years after bilateral vasectomy. J Urol 1939;41:934–40.

11. Gaskill DM, Stewart S, Kirsch WM, et al. Sutureless vasovasostomy: new technique using experimental microclip in rat model. Urology 1992;40:191–4.

12. Gilbert BR, Goldstein M. New directions in male reproductive microsurgery. Microsurgery 1988;9:281–5.

13. Goldstein M. Microspike approximator for vasovasostomy. J Urol 1985;134:74.

14. Goldstein M, Li PS, Matthews GJ. Microsurgical vasovasostomy: the microdot technique of precision suture placement. J Urol 1998;159:188–90.

15. Hagner FR. The operative treatment of sterility in the male. JAMA 1936;107:1851.

16. Hagner FR. Sterility in the male. Surg Gynecol Obstet 1931;52(2A):330–5.

17. Kuang W, Shin PR, Matin S, et al. Initial evaluation of robotic technology for microsurgical vasovasostomy. J Urol 2004;171:300.

18. Lizza EF, Marmar JL, Schmidt SS, et al. Transseptal crossed vasovasostomy. J Urol 1985;134:1131–2.

19. Lynne CM, Carter M, Morris J, et al. Laser-assisted vas anastomosis: a preliminary report. Lasers Surg Med 1983;3:261–3.

20. Marmar JL. Management of the epididymal tubule during an end-to-side vasoepididymostomy. J Urol 1995;154:93–6.

21. Marmar JL. Modified vasoepididymostomy with simultaneous double needle placement, tubulotomy and tubular invagination. J Urol 2000;163:483–6.

22. Massey BD, Nation EF. Vas deferens anastomosis; a report of four consecutive successful cases. J Urol 1949;61:391–5.

23. Moon KH, Bunge RG. Splinted and non-splinted vasovasostomy: experimental study. Invest Urol 1967;5:155–60.

24. O'Conor VJ. Anastomosis of vas deferens after purposeful division for sterility. J Am Med Assoc 1948;136:162.

25. Owen ER. Microsurgical vasovasostomy: a reliable vasectomy reversal. Aust N Z J Surg 1977;47:305–9.

26. Phadke GM, Phadke AG. Experiences in the re-anastomosis of the vas deferens. J Urol 1967;97:888–90.

27. Rolnick HC. Regeneration of the vas deferens. Arch Surg 1924;9:188–203.

28. Rosenbloom D. Reversal of sterility due to vasectomy. Fertil Steril 1956;7:540–5.

29. Schiff J, Li PS, Goldstein M. Robotic microsurgical vasovasostomy and vasoepididymostomy: a prospective randomized study in a rat model. J Urol 2004;171:1720.

30. Silber SJ. Microscopic vasectomy reversal. Fertil Steril 1977;28:1191–202.

31. Silber SJ. Microscopic vasoepididymostomy: specific microanastomosis to the epididymal tubule. Fertil Steril 1978;30:565–71.

32. Silber SJ. Perfect anatomical reconstruction of vas deferens with a new microscopic surgical technique. Fertil Steril 1977;28:72–7.

33. Stefanovic KB, Clark SA, Buncke HJ. Microsurgical epididymovasostomy by tubule intussusception: a new technique in rat model. Fertil Steril 1991;55:189–93.

34. Strauch B. Folding-approximating clamp to simplify microvasovasostomy. Urology 1980;16:295–6.

35. Strode JE. A technique of vasectomy for sterilization. J Urol 1937;37:733–6.

36. Wagenknecht LV, Klosterhalfen H, Schirren C. Microsurgery in andrologic urology. I. Refertilization. J Microsurg 1980;1:370–6.

37. Yarbro ES, Howards SS. Vasovasostomy. Urol Clin North Am1987;14:515–26.

REFERENCES

1. Gugliotta A. "Dr. Sharp with his little knife": therapeutic and punitive origins of eugenic vasectomy—Indiana, 1892–1921. J Hist Med Allied Sci 1998;53:371.

2. Reilly PR. Involuntary sterilization in the United States: a surgical solution. Q Rev Biol 1987;62:153.

3. Sengoopta C. 'Dr Steinach coming to make old young!' Sex glands, vasectomy and the quest for rejuvenation in the roaring twenties. Endeavour 2003;27:122.

4. Ochsner AJ. The surgical treatment of habitual criminals, imbeciles, perverts, paupers, morons, epileptics, and degenerates. Ann Surg 1925;82:321.

5. Drake MJ, Mills IW, Cranston D. On the chequered history of vasectomy. BJU Int 1999;84:475.

6. O'Conor VJ. Anastomosis of vas deferens after purposeful division for sterility. J Am Med Assoc 1948;136:162.

7. Jequier AM. Edward Martin (1859–1938). The founding father of modern clinical andrology. Int J Androl 1991;14:1.

8. Martin E, Carnett JB, Levi JV, et al. The surgical treatment of sterility due to obstruction at the epididymis; together with a study of the morphology of human spermatozoa. Univ Pa Med Bull 1902;15:2.

9. Martin E. Sterility from obstruction cured by operative means. New York Medical Journal 1903;(October 10):1.

10. Martin E. The operation of epididymo-vasostomy for the relief of sterility. Therapeutic Gazette 1909;(December 15):1.

11. Hagner FRIn: Report of two cases of sterility in the male with successful anastomosis between the vas deferens and globus major, vol. 2. New York: The Grafton Press; 1907.

12. Kar JK, Phadke AM. Vaso-epididymal anastomosis. Fertil Steril 1975;26:743.

13. Hagner FR. The operative treatment of sterility in the male. JAMA 1936;107:1851.

14. Bayle H. Masculine sterility, latero-lateral epididymo-deferens anastomosis in azoospermia by obliteration; statistics in 95 surgically explored cases. Urol Cutaneous Rev 1950;54:129.

15. Hanley HG. The surgery of male subfertility; Hunterian lecture delivered at the Royal College of Surgeons of England on 24th May 1955. Ann R Coll Surg Engl 1955;17:159.

16. Rolnick HC. Regeneration of the vas deferens. Arch Surg 1924;9:188.

17. Yarbro ES, Howards SS. Vasovasostomy. Urol Clin North Am 1987;14:515.

18. Hulka JF, Davis JE. Vasectomy and reversible vasocclusion. Fertil Steril 1972;23:683.

19. Getzoff PL. Surgical management of male infertility: results of a survey. Fertil Steril 1973;24:553.

20. Sullivan MJ, Howe GE. Correlation of circulating antisperm antibodies to functional success in vasovasostomy. J Urol 1977;117:189.

21. Requeda E, Charron J, Roberts KD, et al. Fertilizing capacity and sperm antibodies in vasovasostomized men. Fertil Steril 1983;39:197.

22. Schmidt SS. Anastomosis of the vas deferens: an experimental study. II. Successes and failures in experimental anastomosis. J Urol 1959;81:203.

23. Hagan KF, Coffey DS. The adverse effects of sperm during vasovasostomy. J Urol 1977;118:269.

24. Alexander NJ, Schmidt SS. Incidence of antisperm antibody levels and granulomas in men. Fertil Steril 1977;28:655.

25. Silber SJ. Epididymal extravasation following vasectomy as a cause for failure of vasectomy reversal. Fertil Steril 1979;31:309.

26. Schoysman RJ, Bedford JM. The role of the human epididymis in sperm maturation and sperm storage as reflected in the consequences of epididymovasostomy. Fertil Steril 1986;46:293.

27. Amelar RD, Dubin L. Vasectomy reversal. J Urol 1979;121:547.

28. Schmidt SS. Principles of vasovasostomy. Contemp Surg 1975;7:13.

29. Dorsey JW. Surgical correction of post-vasectomy sterility. J Urol 1973;110:554.

30. Schmidt SS. Anastomosis of the vas deferens; an experimental study. I. J Urol 1956;75:300.

31. Fitzpatrick TJ. Vasovasostomy: the flap technique. J Urol 1978;120:78.

32. Singh H, Sharma B. Vasoplasty: flap operation. Br J Urol 1983;55:233.

33. Montie JE, Stewart BH, Levin HS. Intravasal stents for vasovasostomy in canine subjects. Fertil Steril 1973;24:877.

34. Rowland RG, Nanninga JB, O'Conor VJ. Improved results in vasovasostomies using internal plain catgut stents. Urology 1977;10:260.

35. O'Conor VJ Sr. Surgical correction of male sterility. J Urol 1961;85:352.

36. Mehta KC, Ramani PS. A simple technique of re-anastomosis after vasectomy. Br J Urol 1970;42:340.

37. Pai MG, Sampath Kumar BT, Kaundinya C, et al. Vasovasostomy. A clinical study with 10 years' follow-up. Fertil Steril 1973;24:798.

38. Phadke GM, Phadke AG. Experiences in the re-anastomosis of the vas deferens. J Urol 1967;97:888.

39. Roland SI. Splinted and non-splinted vasovasostomy. A review of the literature and a report of nine new cases. Fertil Steril 1961;12:191.

40. Pardanani DS, Kothari ML, Pradhan SA, et al. Surgical restoration of vas continuity after vasectomy: further clinical evaluation of a new operation technique. Fertil Steril 1974;25:319.

41. Silber SJ, Galle J, Friend D. Microscopic vasovasostomy and spermatogenesis. J Urol 1977;117:299.

42. Derrick FC Jr, Yarbrough W, D'Agostino J. Vasovasostomy: results of questionnaire of members of the American Urological Association. J Urol 1973;110:556.

43. Cos LR, Valvo JR, Davis RS, et al. Vasovasostomy: current state of the art. Urology 1983;22:567.

44. Shessel FS, Lynne CM, Politano VA. Use of exteriorized stents in vasovasostomy. Urology 1981;17:163.

45. Belker AM. Urologic microsurgery—current perspectives: I. Vasovasostomy. Urology 1979;14:325.

46. Fernandes M, Shah KN, Draper JW. Vasovasostomy: improved microsurgical technique. J Urol 1968;100: 763.

47. Owen ER. Microsurgical vasovasostomy: a reliable vasectomy reversal. Aust N Z J Surg 1977;47:305.

48. Silber SJ. Microscopic vasectomy reversal. Fertil Steril 1977;28:1191.

49. Silber SJ. Perfect anatomical reconstruction of vas deferens with a new microscopic surgical technique. Fertil Steril 1977;28:72.

50. Ferreiia MC. [Microsurgery of the vas deferens, an experimental study]. AMB Rev Assoc Med Bras 1975;21:243 [in Portuguese].

51. Silber SJ. Microscopic technique for reversal of vasectomy. Surg Gynecol Obstet 1976;143:631.

52. Silber SJ. Microsurgery in clinical urology. Urology 1975;6:150.

53. Silber SJ. Vasectomy and vasectomy reversal. Fertil Steril 1978;29:125.

54. Goldstein M. Microspike approximator for vasovasostomy. J Urol 1985;134:74.

55. Goldstein M, Li PS, Matthews GJ. Microsurgical vasovasostomy: the microdot technique of precision suture placement. J Urol 1998;159:188.

56. Silber SJ, Grotjan HE. Microscopic vasectomy reversal 30 years later: a summary of 4010 cases by the same surgeon. J Androl 2004;25:845.

57. Lee L, McLoughlin MG. Vasovasostomy: a comparison of macroscopic and microscopic techniques at one institution. Fertil Steril 1980;33:54.

58. Boorjian S, Lipkin M, Goldstein M. The impact of obstructive interval and sperm granuloma on outcome of vasectomy reversal. J Urol 2004;171:304.

59. Fuchs EF, Burt RA. Vasectomy reversal performed 15 years or more after vasectomy: correlation of pregnancy outcome with partner age and with pregnancy results of in vitro fertilization with intracytoplasmic sperm injection. Fertil Steril 2002;77:516.

60. Belker AM, Thomas AJ Jr, Fuchs EF, et al. Results of 1,469 microsurgical vasectomy reversals by the Vasovasostomy Study Group. J Urol 1991;145:505.

61. Crain DS, Roberts JL, Amling CL. Practice patterns in vasectomy reversal surgery: results of a questionnaire study among practicing urologists. J Urol 2004;171:311.

62. Schroeder-Printzen I, Diemer T, Weidner W. Vasovasostomy. Urol Int 2003;70:101.

63. Fenster H, McLoughlin MG. Vasovasostomy-microscopy versus macroscopic techniques. Arch Androl 1981;7:201.

64. Fox M. Vasectomy reversal—microsurgery for best results. Br J Urol 1994;73:449.

65. Heidenreich A, Altmann P, Engelmann UH. Microsurgical vasovasostomy versus microsurgical epididymal sperm aspiration/testicular extraction of sperm combined with intracytoplasmic sperm injection. A cost-benefit analysis. Eur Urol 2000;37:609.

66. Lemack GE, Goldstein M. Presence of sperm in the pre-vasectomy reversal semen analysis: incidence and implications. J Urol 1996;155:167.

67. Marmar JL, DeBenedictis TJ, Praiss DE. Use of papaverine during vasovasostomy. Urology 1986; 28:56.

68. Matthews GJ, Schlegel PN, Goldstein M. Patency following microsurgical vasoepididymostomy and vasovasostomy: temporal considerations. J Urol 1995;154:2070.

69. Owen E, Kapila H. Vasectomy reversal. Review of 475 microsurgical vasovasostomies. Med J Aust 1984;140:398.

70. Rothman I, Berger RE, Cummings P, et al. Randomized clinical trial of an absorbable stent for vasectomy reversal. J Urol 1997;157:1697.

71. Silber SJ. Pregnancy after vasovasostomy for vasectomy reversal: a study of factors affecting long-term return of fertility in 282 patients followed for 10 years. Hum Reprod 1989;4:318.

72. Weiske WH. Ergebnisse bei 376 Refertilisie-rungsoperationen nach zwei Jahren. Urologe A 1997; 37(Suppl):567 [in German].

73. Yamamoto M, Hibi H, Yokoi K, et al. Surgical outcome of microscopic vasectomy reversal: an analysis of 30 cases. Nagoya J Med Sci 1997;60:37.

74. Weinerth JL. Long-term management of vasovasostomy patients. Fertil Steril 1984;41:625.

75. Willscher MK, Novicki DE. Simplified technique for microscopic vasovasostomy. Urology 1980;15:147.

76. Wright GM, Cato A, Webb DR. Microsurgical vasovasostomy in military personnel. Aust N Z J Surg 1995;65:20.

77. Fischer MA, Grantmyre JE. Comparison of modified one- and two-layer microsurgical vasovasostomy. BJU Int 2000;85:1085.

78. Lee HY. A 20-year experience with vasovasostomy. J Urol 1986;136:413.

79. Schoysman R. Delay of appearance of spermatozoa in the ejaculate after vaso-epididymostomy e vasovasostomy. Acta Eur Fertil 1990;21:125.

80. Sharlip ID. Vasovasostomy: comparison of two microsurgical techniques. Urology 1981;17:347.

81. Hartig PR, Meyer JJ. Vasovasostomy with use of intraoperative vasography. Urology 1982;19:404.

82. Paulson DF, Lindsey CM, Anderson EE. Simplified technique for vasography. Fertil Steril 1974;25:906.

83. Jenkins IL, Blacklock NJ. Reversal of vasectomy. Int J Gynaecol Obstet 1979;17:144.

84. Thomas AJ Jr. Vasoepididymostomy. Urol Clin North Am 1987;14:527.

85. Lespinasse VD. Obstructive sterility in the male. Treatment by direct vaso-epididymostomy. JAMA 1918;70:448.

86. Silber SJ. Microscopic vasoepididymostomy: specific microanastomosis to the epididymal tubule. Fertil Steril 1978;30:565.

87. Silber SJ. Vasoepididymostomy to the head of the epididymis: recovery of normal spermatozoal motility. Fertil Steril 1980;34:149.

88. Wagenknecht LV, Klosterhalfen H, Schirren C. Microsurgery in andrologic urology. I. Refertilization. J Microsurg 1980;1:370.

89. Berger RE. Triangulation end-to-side vasoepididymostomy. J Urol 1998;159:1951.

90. Chan PT, Li PS, Goldstein M. Microsurgical vasoepididymostomy: a prospective randomized study of 3 intussusception techniques in rats. J Urol 2003;169:1924.

91. Pavlovich CP, Schlegel PN. Fertility options after vasectomy: a cost-effectiveness analysis. Fertil Steril 1997;67:133.

92. Kolettis PN, Thomas AJ Jr. Vasoepididymostomy for vasectomy reversal: a critical assessment in the era of intracytoplasmic sperm injection. J Urol 1997;158:467.

93. Rosemberg SK, Elson L, Nathan LE Jr. Carbon dioxide laser microsurgical vasovasostomy. Urology 1985;25:53.

94. Trickett RI, Wang D, Maitz P, et al. Laser welding of vas deferens in rodents: initial experience with fluid solders. Microsurgery 1998;18:414.

95. Gaskill DM, Stewart S, Kirsch WM, et al. Sutureless vasovasostomy: new technique using experimental microclip in rat model. Urology 1992;40:191.

96. Silverstein JI, Mellinger BC. Fibrin glue vasal anastomosis compared to conventional sutured vasovasostomy in the rat. J Urol 1991;145:1288.

97. Weiss JN, Mellinger BC. Fertility rates with delayed fibrin glue: vasovasostomy in rats. Fertil Steril 1992;57:908.

98. Schiff J, Li PS, Goldstein M. Toward a sutureless vasovasostomy: use of biomaterials and surgical sealants in a rodent vasovasostomy model. J Urol 2004;172:1192.

99. Schiff J, Li PS, Goldstein M. Robotic microsurgical vasovasostomy and vasoepididymostomy: a prospective randomized study in a rat model. J Urol 2004;171:1720.

Techniques for Vasectomy Reversal

Larry I. Lipshultz, MD*, Jon A. Rumohr, MD, Richard C. Bennett, MD

KEYWORDS

- Vasectomy • Reversal • Techniques • Methods
- Vasovasostomy • Epididymovasostomy
- Vasoepididymostomy

Urologists perform approximately 500,000 vasectomies in the United States each year.[1] Because of changing social circumstances, however, up to 6% of men request reversal after vasectomy.[2] Microsurgical reconstruction also may be requested for other, less common sources of vasal occlusion such as iatrogenic injury (hernia repair), secondary obstruction caused by infections, and postvasectomy pain syndrome (PVPS). Vasovasostomy (VV) and epididymovasostomy (EV) are thus commonly requested procedures for the urologist. The regularity with which this operation is requested and performed, however, belies its degree of difficulty and the nuances associated with treating couples desiring fertility. This article details the contemporary preoperative preparation, microsurgical techniques, and postoperative care recommended for vasectomy reversal. The two-layer VV and intussuscepted EV techniques are presented in detail.

PREPARATION FOR VASECTOMY REVERSAL
Specialized Training

It generally is accepted that microsurgical vasectomy reversal yields better results than macrosurgical anastomoses.[3] Therefore, requisite training in microsurgical techniques is recommended. The importance of the surgeon's microsurgical expertise is particularly relevant when an EV is indicated. Although preoperative nomograms have been advocated by some to aid in predicting the need for an EV versus a VV, certain men who have favorable preoperative parameters nonetheless will require the more technically demanding EV.[4]

Consequently, a vasectomy reversal ideally is performed by a surgeon prepared to perform both VVs and EVs as dictated by intraoperative findings. The surgeon should discuss the differences between these techniques and the expected outcomes and the surgeon's own experience.

Patient Evaluation

A thorough preoperative history of the male and female partner is taken, and a focused physical examination of the male is performed. By far, the most important prognostic factor for reversal success is the duration of occlusion.[2,3] A detailed history of the patient's vasectomy, including a postvasectomy hematoma or infection can prepare the surgeon for peri-testicular inflammatory changes and a more difficult dissection and reanastomosis. The surgeon should attempt to identify other historical factors that may impact on the surgical procedures such as previous inguinal surgery (especially hernia repairs using mesh after vasectomy), prior proven male fertility, and his general medical conditions. On physical examination, prognostic factors include the presence of a sperm granuloma[5] and the testicular vasal segment[6] length, both of which may act to decompress the epididymis and may prevent concurrent epididymal obstruction. Large missing vasal segments, testicular abnormalities, and marked induration of the vas deferens or epididymis should be noted. Serum follicle-stimulating hormone (FSH) testing is unnecessary before most reconstructions, unless small testes are

Division of Male Reproductive Medicine and Surgery, Scott Department of Urology, Baylor College of Medicine, 6560 Fannin, Suite 2100, Houston, TX 77030, USA
* Corresponding author.
E-mail address: larryl@bcm.edu (L.I. Lipshultz).

Urol Clin N Am 36 (2009) 375–382
doi:10.1016/j.ucl.2009.05.011

noted on examination, and testicular damage is suspected.

Patients or couples interested in pursuing vasectomy reversal to restore fertility should be apprised of the risks, benefits and alternatives to surgical reconstruction. Realistic, patient-specific operative outcomes using preoperative nomograms and the surgeon's own outcome data can be useful in this setting.[3,7] In addition, the reproductive potential of the female partner should be assessed and discussed objectively with the couple. This is particularly important if the woman is nulliparous or over 35 years of age. Including the woman's gynecologist in this workup helps establish an unbiased assessment of the female partner's fertility potential.

The surgeon should be prepared to present alternatives to vasectomy reversal, including the extraction of sperm for in vitro fertilization (IVF) with ICSI, donor sperm insemination, and adoption. Additionally, the potential and desirability of a multiple-gestation pregnancy with assisted reproduction should be taken into account. The cost of multiple pregnancies using IVF with ICSI is significantly greater than that of vasectomy reversal.[8]

If vasectomy reversal is to be performed, the option of intraoperative sperm cryopreservation, if available, should be considered. Sperm may be harvested from the testicular vasal segment, from an incised epididymal tubule, or from the testicle (TESE) at the time of reconstruction. There is debate among practitioners as to the cost-effectiveness and utility of sperm cryopreservation, with some advocating and others discouraging its practice.[9,10] The authors' practice is to encourage cryopreservation if preoperative parameters predict EV and if the patient would be unwilling to undergo further procedures for IVF with ICSI in the event of a failed reconstruction. This also may allow couples to pursue IVF concurrently with reconstruction.

Instrumentation and Equipment

The microsurgical instrumentation required for vasectomy reversal should be customized for each individual surgeon's hands and technique. Various microsurgical instruments are available from numerous companies. The microsurgical instrument set that the authors find essential to performing vasectomy reversal are outlined in **Table 1**. It is important to have duplicates of these instruments if contamination or malfunction occurs during the case.

Various sutures are available for microsurgical cases. The suture preference of the authors is 10-0 nylon 2XBRM5 double-armed for luminal VV stitches and the open epididymal tubule-to-vas lumen during an EV. A 9-0 nylon HSV6 suture is used for the seromuscular layer of the VV, and for the epididymal tunical edge to the seromuscular vas (EV).

The patient is positioned supine, on a surgical bed with a central support and leg extension (Skytron). Comfortable positioning is important for the surgeon and patient during a potentially lengthy procedure. The operative microscope used by the authors is a Zeiss model ZMS-414. A microscope, preferably with phase contrast, is needed in the operating room for the intraoperative examination of the vasal or epididymal fluid.

Anesthetic Considerations

The anesthetic used for vasectomy reversal is surgeon- and patient-dependant. Surgeons comfortable with the combination of local anesthetic and sedation use a one-to-one mixture of 1% lidocaine HCl and 0.25% bupivacaine HCl with intravenous sedation. General anesthesia or epidural have significant advantages, including:

- For a highly anxious patient
- Surgeon preference

Table 1		
Microsurgical instruments		
3.3 Bishop Harmon Forceps	#5 Jeweler's Forceps	Vannasd Pattern Suture Scissors
McPherson tying forceps	Curved Castroviejo needle holder, nonlocking	Nerve holder (#4)
0.12 Castroviejo suturing forceps	12 cm Halsey needle holder	Towel clamps
Jacobson mosquito forceps	Straight Iris scissors	#3 knife handle
#3 Jeweler's forceps (2)	Vannas pattern dissecting scissors	Dennis blade holder

- If the expected procedure length is longer than 3 hours
- If extensive mobilization of the vas or epididymis is anticipated.

MICROSCOPIC VASOVASOSTOMY
Preparation and Exposure

After induction of general anesthesia, the patient is shaved and prepared for standard surgery. The authors have found a layer of waterproof drapes useful to avoid soaking the patient with irrigation. The groin is included in the operative field for an extended incision, if necessary, and the penis draped cephalad to avoid interference. The operating microscope is positioned at head of the bed, on the patient's left, and the surgeon is seated with his dominant hand toward the foot. The operating table is slid to the foot (certain tables will require a leg extension or support), permitting comfortable seating for the surgeon and assistant. The authors deliver the testes and spermatic cords with the tunica vaginalis intact through vertical, paramedian scrotal incisions.

A ball tip towel clamp is placed around the vas deferens and adventitia on the testicular side of the vasectomy site, and downward traction is applied. Curved iris scissors are passed behind the vas, and the assistant places a Jacobson mosquito in this space. Minimal dissection of the vasal adventitia at this site is performed, with care to leave abundant peri-vasal blood supply. A 5-0 chromic stay suture is placed through the adventitia of the vas 1 to 2 cm inferior to the anticipated transection site. It is important to minimize the use of cautery, using only a microtip bipolar at low setting if necessary. A 2 to 3 mm slotted nerve holder then is placed on the vas at the selected transection site; an Adson or other toothed forceps grasps the vasectomy site to provide stability, and a Dennis blade is passed briskly through the slot. The vas should be under no tension during the transection to avoid protrusion of the mucosal edge. The abdominal vas deferens is isolated and divided in an identical manner. The intervening vasal segment is ligated at each end with a 4-0 chromic tie, or excised. Bleeding is controlled with the microtip bipolar device, taking care to minimize contact with the vas itself. At this point, instillation of saline or methylene blue using an angiocatheter into the lumen of the abdominal vas may be performed. Back pressure or an absence of blue tint in a catheterized urine sample suggests obstruction. The authors do not perform this maneuver routinely, unless the patient's prior history suggests obstruction.

Attention next is turned to the fluid expressed from the testicular vas. Fluid may flow freely from the lumen, or may require gentle pressure on the epididymis and milking of the convoluted vas. The quality and quantity of the fluid are noted. The fluid is aspirated with a 3 mL syringe fitted with a 25 French angiocatheter, primed with 0.1 cc of either human tubular fluid (HTF) or normal saline. The former fluid is preferred if cryopreservation is a consideration. The lumen may be dilated gently with a fine jeweler's forceps to facilitate the aspiration. A drop of the aspirated fluid then is examined under 400 × magnification. Whole sperm and the degree of sperm motility, sperm parts, or a blizzard effect of degenerated cells may be observed. The decision to perform a VV or EV is based in large part on the macro- and microscopic quality of the fluid. This is discussed elsewhere in this article. If motile sperm are observed and cryopreservation desired, continuous gentle pressure is applied to the epididymis/convoluted vas, and the fluid is collected by the assistant until the flow ceases. The fluid is stored in sperm-safe containers sterilized by radiation and sent to the laboratory for cryopreservation. Prior coordination with laboratory personnel is critical for proper preparation and preservation for later use with ICSI, if necessary.

If the fluid expressed from the testicular vas deferens is suitable for VV, the two vasal ends are approximated. There are several methods to approximate the two ends of the vas at this point. Some surgeons use a vas approximating clamp, while others, including the authors, prefer an adventitial holding stitch. Regardless of technique, it is important to ensure that the ends overlap easily and that the anastomosis will be under no tension. The authors place a 5-0 PDS suture through the loose adventitia of each vasal end, with attention paid to symmetry. If the approximating suture is asymmetrical, the cut ends of the vas will not be in an ideal position for anastomosis. As the assistant ties the 5-0 approximating suture, the surgeon crosses over the previously placed chromic stay sutures to approximate the vasa until the 5-0 PDS is tied securely. Scott elastic retractor hooks secured to the drapes are particularly useful at this point to expose the approximated vasal ends and to minimize encroaching scrotal or spermatic cord fat.

The authors then perform a two-layer vasovasostomy. The 6 o'clock position on each vas is identified with a micropoint marker. The anastomosis begins with interrupted 9-0 nylon stitches (Sharpoint, half-circle needle) at the 5 o'clock,

6 o'clock, and 7 o'clock positions through the vasal muscularis and adventitia (**Fig. 1**). An interrupted 10-0 nylon suture (Sharpoint, biconcave needle) then is passed through the mucosal layer at the 6 o'clock position, being sure to include a small of bite of muscularis (**Fig. 2**). A drop of methylene blue placed on the cut surface of the vas improves visualization of the mucosal surface. Additional mucosal sutures are placed on either side of this stitch and tied down. Three to five additional mucosal stitches then are placed equidistant from each other, and left untied until all are placed (**Fig. 3**). The mucosal sutures then are tied down sequentially. A 9-0 nylon suture is placed though the seromuscular layer at the 12 o'clock position. Interrupted seromuscular 9-0 nylon sutures then are placed circumferentially to complete the anastomosis (**Fig. 4**).

A modified, single-layer technique for VV has been described. Proponents of the technique find it simpler, more expeditious, and note that it may not require an operating microscope. In small, single-surgeon series, the results of this technique have compared favorably with the two-layer technique in terms of patency and pregnancy rates.[11] A truly randomized study of the modified microscopic single-layer versus two-layer VV, performed by surgeons facile in both techniques, has not been reported, however.

Postoperative care

A gentle pressure dressing and scrotal support are placed when the operation is complete. An ice pack can be applied intermittently for 24 hours after surgery, and scrotal supporters or briefs are encouraged for 2 weeks. Light physical activity is suggested for the 3-week interval after reversal, and patients are encouraged to abstain from

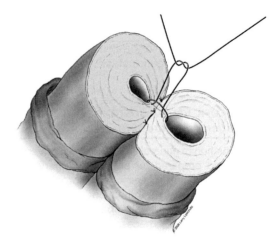

Fig. 2. A 6 o'clock 10-0 nylon suture is placed and tied down, followed by additional 4 o'clock and 8 o'clock sutures. (*Courtesy of* Larry I. Lipshultz, MD, Houston, TX; with permission).

sexual activity for 2 weeks. Oral analgesics are adequate for pain control. Patients return for a semen analysis at 6 weeks, and every 3 months thereafter for 1 year. Anecdotally, the author has found a 30-day course of nonsteroidal anti-inflammatory drugs (NSAIDs) or a short steroid taper may benefit those patients with early severe oligospermia or asthenospermia in whom intraoperative findings were predictive of a more positive outcome.

Complications of vasectomy reversal are uncommon. Scrotal hematoma, the most serious adverse event, is avoided with meticulous

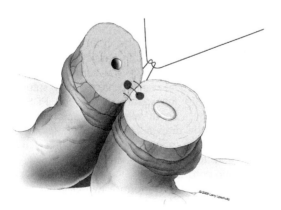

Fig. 1. Three interrupted posterior seromuscular layer 9-0 nylon sutures are placed initially. (*Courtesy of* Larry I. Lipshultz, MD, Houston, TX; with permission).

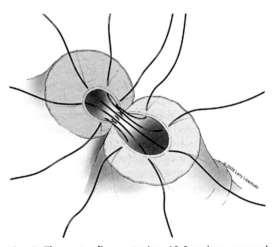

Fig. 3. Three to five anterior 10-0 nylon mucosal sutures are placed first, then tied down sequentially. (*Courtesy of* Larry I. Lipshultz, MD, Houston, TX; with permission).

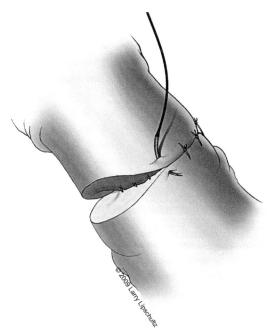

Fig. 4. Additional circumferential 9-0 nylon seromuscular layer sutures are placed to complete the anastomosis. (*Courtesy of* Larry I. Lipshultz, MD, Houston, TX; with permission).

hemostasis throughout the dissection. Hematomas, should they arise, should be evacuated and drained to minimize the effect of local inflammatory mediators on the still-fragile anastomosis. Wound infections are rare in the era of perioperative antibiotics, but should be treated in an appropriately aggressive manner. The testicular blood supply is avoided easily and spared during reversal, but verification of arterial patency can be aided with intraoperative micro-Doppler ultrasound (Vascular Technology, Incorporated) in complicated reconstructions.

VASOEPIDIDYMOSTOMY

An epididymovasostomy is performed when deemed necessary by the intraoperative fluid examination. When an EV is considered, the tunica vaginalis is opened and the testicle and epididymis exposed. The epididymis is grasped between the thumb and forefinger. Inspections of the epididymis under magnification may reveal a point of demarcation, with dilated tubules proximal to the obstruction. A ruptured tubule caused by back pressure after vasectomy may be the cause of epididymal obstruction.[12] The location for the EV should be as distal as possible in the epididymis. The more intact epididymis that can be preserved, the more time the sperm will

have in the epididymis to mature and gain motility. Therefore, the epididymal tunic is opened caudally and progress made toward the caput until sperm is identified in the epididymal fluid from a single isolated tubule. A 0.5 cm opening is made in the tunic of the epididymis with microdissecting scissors. A dilated tubule then is identified and dissected free of the surrounding tissue. Methylene blue or indigo carmine irrigation provides better visualization of the tissue planes and tubules.

Once a suitable tubule it identified visually, the first sutures are placed. The needle of a 10-0 double armed suture is passed through the tubular wall at the 2 o'clock position. A needle from a second 10-0 double armed suture then is passed at the 10 o'clock position. These needles are not pulled all the way through the wall of the tubule. Instead, they are left in the wall and rotated laterally, to allow for incision of the tubule between the needles. A 20 gauge V-lance knife (Alcon Surgical) then is used to make a 0.5 mm puncture between the two needles of the 10-0 sutures (**Fig. 5**). The 10-0 sutures then can be advanced the rest of the way through the wall of the tubule. Care must be taken to not inadvertently pull out these sutures before the intussusception.

The fluid from this tubule is sampled carefully with an aspirating syringe and a 22 gauge angiocatheter. The fluid is examined under phase microscopy in the operating room, to ensure sperm are identified. If the patient expressed a desire to bank sperm, motile sperm identified in the epididymal fluid can be collected for cryopreservation. If whole sperm are identified, but none are motile, a TESE for cryopreservation can

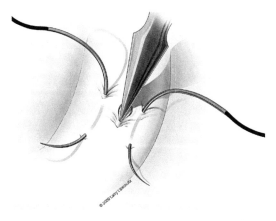

Fig. 5. Epididimoty is made between the parallel needles of the 10-0 sutures. (*Courtesy of* Larry I. Lipshultz, MD, Houston, TX; with permission).

be performed at the end of the procedure. If sperm are identified in the effluxing epididymal fluid, the surgeon can proceed with the EV. If no sperm are identified, a new tunical opening is made more proximally, and the process is repeated.

The abdominal vas then must be tunneled through the tunica vaginalis of the testicle. Sufficient length of abdominal vas must be mobilized to reach the epididymis. This may require extension of the original incision toward the groin to better expose the vas. The vas should be left with as much adventitia as possible to ensure adequate blood supply to the anastomosis. A 5-0 PDS suture then is placed at the adventitial base of the mobilized abdominal vas segment. A Jacobson mosquito is used to make a puncture opening within the tunica vaginalis, through which the 5-0 PDS adventitial suture and the vas are pulled.

The 5-0 PDS then can be used to anchor the vas to the tunical covering of the epididymis. The needle of the 5-0 PDS is passed through the edge of the tunica on the epididymis and then tied down. It is important to ensure that the cut end of the vas is aligned properly with the opened epididymal tubule before tying down the PDS (**Fig. 6**). A 7-0 nonabsorbable suture then can be sutured through the tunica of the epididymis midway between the PDS and the opened tubule. Placing this 7-0 suture through the corresponding location on the outer wall of the vas and tying it down will allow for better support and alignment of the vas and tubule. 9-0 nylon interrupted sutures then are placed between the edge of epididymal tunic

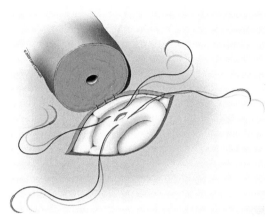

Fig. 7. Vas defrens sutured to the tunical covering of the epididymis. The epididymal sutures are aligned with the lumen of the vas defrens. (*Courtesy of* Larry I. Lipshultz, MD, Houston, TX; with permission).

and seromuscular layer of the vas (**Fig. 7**). The double-armed 10-0 sutures now are used to create an intussuscepted anastomosis. The needles are passed inside-out through the vasal lumen. This is done in a near-near, far-far fashion (**Fig. 8**). The two needles on the same side of the luminal opening as the vas are passed through the inferior edge of the vasal lumen at the 4 o'clock and 8 o'clock positions. The sutures on the opposite site of the tubular opening are passed at the 10 o'clock and 2 o'clock positions. When done properly, the loops created by the 10-0 suture are visible between the vas and tubal before tying down the sutures. A loose surgeon's knot is thrown in both sutures before tensioning the sutures. The assistant uses a jeweler's forceps to bring the vas down to the tubule, while the first and then second sutures are tied down. Additional 9-0 sutures then are used to complete the outer

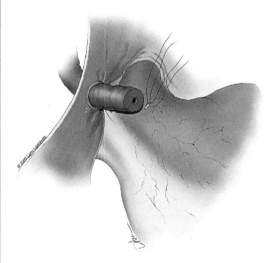

Fig. 6. Abdominal vas defrens is tunneled through the tunica vaginalis. (*Courtesy of* Larry I. Lipshultz, MD, Houston, TX; with permission).

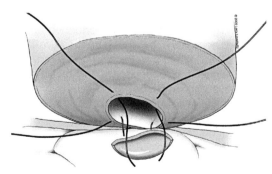

Fig. 8. The 10-0 sutures are placed through the lumen of the vas defrens for the intussuscepted anastomosis. (*Courtesy of* Larry I. Lipshultz, MD, Houston, TX; with permission).

layer of sutures from the epididymal tunic to the seromuscular vas.

The tunica vaginalis then is closed over the testicle and the epididymis, with a running 3-0 chromic suture. The testicle is placed back within the scrotum. The dartos layer is closed with a running 3-0 chromic suture, and the skin with interrupted horizontal mattress sutures.

Postoperative care is similar to that following a VV, although some surgeons may recommend a longer period of abstinence.

INTRAOPERATIVE CONSIDERATIONS AND SUCCESS RATE

The success rate of vasectomy reversal depends upon the time interval from vasectomy to reversal, the intraoperative findings, and the subsequent procedure chosen. The Vasovasostomy Study Group showed a 97% patency rate and 76% pregnancy rate following VV in patients less than 3 years out from vasectomy. These rates fall as the interval increases, with a patency rate of 71% and pregnancy rate of 30% at greater than

15 years.[13] Other studies have not shown a direct correlation between time interval and success, but have observed significantly lower success rates after a 15-year time interval between vasectomy and reversal.[5]

Intraoperatively, the fluid from the testicular side of the transected vas deferens may be graded 1 to 5 (**Box 1**).[13]

The success rates based upon fluid grade were outlined by the Vasovasostomy Study Group in 1991 (**Table 2**).

The pregnancy rate and likelihood that sperm will be present in the ejaculate are higher when the vasal fluid appears watery (colorless, transparent, clear) or cloudy. If the fluid is thick and creamy, the rates diminish.[2] The overall success rate for VV is good with fluid grades 1 to 4; however some experienced microsurgeons prefer to perform a vasoepididymostomy if grade 4 or 5 fluid is found.[14]

The technique of EV has evolved over time. Original procedures were performed in an end-to-end fashion. Later, the end-to-side anastomosis became popular, which was refined further to the current two or three suture intussusception techniques. Published patency rates for the current techniques of intussuscepted end-to-side EV are 80% to 85% with pregnancy rates of 40% to 45%.[15–17]

The surgical techniques outlined herein represent the preferences of the authors. There are multiple other established and experimental techniques for vasectomy reversal. The technique of EV has evolved over the years. The two- and three-suture intussusception techniques have been shown to be comparable or superior to end-to-side EV techniques: with fewer late failures.[17] Further investigation and validation of new surgical techniques and their outcomes are essential to the continued advancement in the field of microsurgical vasectomy reversal.

Table 2
Vasovasectomy study group success rates

Quality of Sperm	Return of Sperm to the Ejaculate (%)	Pregnancy Rate (%)
Grade 1	94	63
Grade 2	91	54
Grade 3	96	50
Grade 4	75	44
Grade 5	60	31

From Belker AM, Thomas AJ, Fuchs EF, et al. Results of 1469 microsurgical vasectomy reversals by the Vasovasostomy Study Group. J Urol 1991;145:505–11; with permission.

REFERENCES

1. Pryor JL, Schow DA. Vasectomy. In: Graham SD, Glenn JF, editors. Glenn's urologic surgery. 5th edition. Philadelphia: Lippincott Williams & Wilkins; 1998. p. 487–92.

2. Potts JM, Pasqualotto FF, Nelson D, et al. Patient characteristics associated with vasectomy reversal. J Urol 1999;161(6):1835–9.

3. Belker AM. Microsurgical vasectomy reversal. In: Lytton B, Catalona WJ, Lipshultz LI, editors. Advances in urology. Chicago: Year Book Medical; 1988. p. 193–230.

4. Parekattil SJ, Kuang W, Agarwal A, et al. Model to predict if a vasoepidimostomy will be required for vasectomy reversal. J Urol 2005;173(5): 1681–4.

5. Boorjian S, Lipkin M, Goldstein M. The impact of obstructive interval and granuloma on outcome of vasectomy reversal. J Urol 2004;171(1):304–6.

6. Witt M, Heron S, Lipshultz LI. The postvasectomy length of the testicular vasal remnant: a predictor of surgical outcome in microscopic vasectomy reversal. J Urol 1994;151(4):892–4.

7. Fenig DM, Kattan MW, et al. Presented at Annual meeting, AUA, 2008.

8. Meng MV, Greene KL, Turek PJ. Surgery of assisted reproduction? A decision analysis of treatment costs in male infertility. J Urol 2005;174(5): 1926–31.

9. Glazier DB, Marmar JL, Mayer E, et al. The fate of cryopreserved sperm acquired during vasectomy reversals. J Urol 1999;161(2):463–6.

10. Boyle KE, Thomas AJ Jr, Marmar JL, et al. Sperm harvesting and cryopreservation during vasectomy reversal is not cost-effective. Fertil Steril 2006; 85(4):961–4.

11. Fischer MA, Grantmyre JE. Comparison of modified one- and two-layer microsurgical vasovasostomy. BJU Int 2000;85(9):1085–8.

12. Silber SJ. Epididymal extravasation following vasectomy as a cause for failure of vasectomy reversal. Fertil Steril 1979;31:309–15.

13. Belker AM, Thomas AJ, Fuchs EF, et al. Results of 1,469 microsurgical vasectomy reversals by the vasovasostomy study group. J Urol 1991;145:505–11.

14. Kolettis PN, Burns JR, Nangia AK, et al. Outcomes for vasovasostomy performed when only sperm parts are present in the vasal fluid. J Androl 2006;27:565–7.

15. Kolettis PN, Thomas JR. Vasoepididymostomy for vasectomy reversal: a critical assessment in the era of intracytoplasmic sperm injection. J Urol 1997;158:467–70.

16. Chan PT, Brandell RA, Goldstein M. Prospective analysis of outcomes after microsurgical intussusception vasoepididymostomy. Br J Urol 2005;96:598–601.

17. Schiff J, Chan P, Li P, et al. Outcome and late failures compared in 4 techniques of microsurgical vasoepididymostomy in 153 consecutive men. J Urol 2005; 174:651–5.

Factors Predicting Successful Microsurgical Vasectomy Reversal

Harris M. Nagler, MD, FACS[a,b,c,*], Howard Jung, MD[b]

KEYWORDS

- Vasectomy reversal • Vasovasostomy
- Vasoepididymostomy • Predictive factors
- Infertility

A man who desires restoration of fertility after vasectomy has two main treatment options for having his genetic child: vasectomy reversal or sperm extraction with subsequent in vitro fertilization with intracytoplasmic sperm injection (IVF-ICSI). Other options for parenting include donor sperm or adoption. Microsurgical reconstructive techniques and their widespread availability have made vasectomy reversal a realistic option for many couples. However, the technical and functional success of these reconstructive procedures, reported as patency and pregnancy rates, respectively, are varied. Studies on vasovasostomy (VV) outcomes report patency rates between 75% and 86% and pregnancy rates between 45% and 70%.[1–6] Studies on vasoepididymostomy (VE) outcomes report patency rates between 31% and 92% and pregnancy rates between 10% and 50%.[7–23] Because couples have a variety of options for parenting, it would be helpful to identify factors that predict the outcome of attempted reconstruction for an individual.

Vasectomy reversal outcomes are varied because there are many factors that alter the chance of success. Some of these factors become known preoperatively, whereas others can only be ascertained at the time of surgery. Preoperatively, the urologist must identify and understand the predictive value of these factors in order to properly advise the patient and his partner. The discussion with the couple should include a comparison of their likelihood of success with vasectomy reversal compared to their likelihood of success with testicular sperm extraction, which yields 100% successful sperm retrieval rates in cases of obstructive azoospermia, and subsequent IVF-ICSI, which yields 20% to 37% pregnancy rates per initiated cycle, as per the most recently published report from the Centers for Disease Control in 2005.[24] Intraoperatively, the urologist must identify factors and understand how they will affect the decision to proceed to a VE. The significance of postoperative management is unclear; nevertheless, it deserves consideration. This article systematically reviews each of these phases of decision-making and management.

PREOPERATIVE FACTORS
Obstructive Interval

The impact of increasing obstructive interval on the success of vasectomy reversal was first reported by Silber.[3] Although Silber reported that there was a precipitous decrease in success 10 years after vasectomy, this tenet was initially challenged by the Vasovasostomy Study Group.[1] This

[a] The Albert Einstein College of Medicine of Yeshiva University, 1300 Morris Park Avenue, Bronx, NY 10461, USA
[b] Sol and Margaret Berger Department of Urology, Beth Israel Medical Center, 10 Union Square East, Suite 3A, New York, NY 10003, USA
[c] Academic Affairs/Graduate Medical Education, Beth Israel Medical Center, 10 Union Square East, Suite 3A, New York, NY 10003, USA
* Corresponding author. Sol and Margaret Berger Department of Urology, Beth Israel Medical Center, 10 Union Square East, Suite 3A, New York, NY 10003.
E-mail address: hnagler@chpnet.org (H.M. Nagler).

Urol Clin N Am 36 (2009) 383–390
doi:10.1016/j.ucl.2009.05.010

landmark work demonstrated that there is not a precipitous decline in success at any point of time after vasectomy, but, rather, a gradual downward trend (**Fig. 1**). In contrast, a more recent study from Boorjian and colleagues[5] demonstrated no change in patency rates (88%–91%), even 15 years after vasectomy. These investigators noted that the pregnancy rates declined precipitously 15 years after vasectomy, from 82% to 89%, to 44%; however, before 15 years they stayed the same, even when a more complicated VE was performed. The investigators attributed their higher overall success rates to newer reconstructive techniques and their higher VE success rates to routine use of VE in cases of intravasal azoospermia (unless there was clear, copious fluid). It is important to note that a pregnancy rate of 44% in patients 15 years after vasectomy is still higher than reported pregnancy rates of 20% to 37% per IVF-ICSI cycle. Kolettis and colleagues[25] determined outcomes for vasectomy reversal after at least 10 years of obstruction. The patency/pregnancy rate for obstructive interval of 10 to 15, 16 to 19, and 20 or more years was 74%/40%, 87%/36%, and 75%/27%, respectively. When compared to IVF-ICSI rates contemporaneous to this article (25% per initiated cycle in 2002),[26] vasectomy reversal still yielded higher success rates.

Currently, pregnancy rates are used to compare success between IVF-ICSI and vasectomy reversal. Malizia and colleagues[27] proposed cumulative live-birth rates over six cycles of IVF as a more appropriate measure of success because it represents achievement of the ultimate goal, the birth of a live child, after completed treatment. In their series of 6,164 patients undergoing 14,248 cycles, they demonstrated overall cumulative live-birth rates between 51% and 72% that was age-dependent (65%–86% in females <40 years old and 23%–42% in females >39 years old). Note that these success rates are for IVF overall, and are not specific to cases that used ICSI. Future discussion of cumulative live-birth rates as an outcome should compare rates specific to IVF-ICSI after sperm extraction and live-birth rates at any point in time after a vasectomy reversal.

In addition to its adverse effect on success of VV, increasing obstructive interval is also associated with an increased incidence of epididymal obstruction and the resultant need for VE. Although Boorjian and colleagues[5] reported a 25% overall incidence of VE in their series, with no significant difference in use according to obstructive interval, Fuchs and Burt[28] reported that 62% of patients with an obstructive interval 15 years or more required a VE for repair. Parekattil and colleagues[29] designed a mathematical computer model based on obstructive interval and patient age to detect the need for a VE. This model was 100% sensitive and 58.8% specific

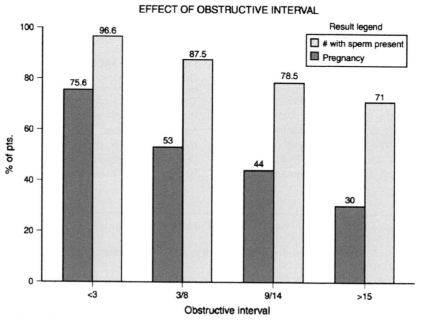

Fig. 1. Increasing intervals of obstruction show a gradual downward trend in success rates of reconstruction. (*From* Belker AM, Thomas AJ, Fuchs EF, et al. Results of 1,469 microsurgical vasectomy reversals by the Vasovasostomy Study Group. J Urol 1991;145:507; with permission.)

with an area under the receiver-operating curve of 0.8. This model was subsequently validated to have 84% sensitivity and 58% specificity in a total of 345 patients at seven institutions.[30] These studies highlight a clear relationship between obstructive interval and epididymal obstruction requiring a more complicated and less successful VE for repair.

Prior Fertility

Nearly all patients undergoing vasectomy reversal have a history of having previously fathered children or impregnated a partner.[31] Although a history of fertility does not ensure normal spermatogenesis, the absence of previous fertility should raise concern. The vasectomy patient without prior fertility should undergo the standard endocrinologic infertility evaluation; however, it should be noted that the incidence of clinically significant endocrinopathies in infertile men is low (1.7%). Routine endocrinologic evaluation is not generally required in the individual with normal testicular size, consistency, and history of fertility prior to vasectomy.[32]

Prior fertility in the female partner may provide additional useful information. There is a statistically significant difference between pregnancy rates after vasectomy reversal for patients whose current spouse was previously pregnant (57%) and those whose current spouse had not been previously pregnant (49%).[1]

Prior Inguinal Surgery

Inguinal surgery, usually a pediatric hernia repair or a hernia repair with mesh, may result in a second point of vasal obstruction. The true prevalence of vasal obstruction from inguinal surgery is not known; however, in a multi-institutional report, 14 men were found to have vasal obstruction after hernia repair with mesh: 9 had bilateral obstruction and 5 had unilateral obstruction with contralateral testis atrophy or epididymal obstruction.[33] The potential significance of this should be reviewed with the patient before reconstruction is attempted. Repair of obstruction in the inguinal canal or retroperitoneum can be technically demanding. Laparoscopy has been used for retrieval and mobilization of a retroperitoneal vas deferens in order to permit a tension-free, patent anastomosis in a case of extensive mesh-induced fibrosis of the inguinal vas deferens after herniorrhaphy.[34] Furthermore, the need to complete two anastomoses on the same vas may result in a devascularized segment and technical failure.

Lizza and colleagues[35] reviewed the records of 11 patients undergoing transseptal-crossed VV

for obstructive azoospermia resulting from unilateral vasal obstruction and damage to the contralateral testis. They reported 50% patency rates and 25% pregnancy rates. Sabanegh and Thomas[36] reported similar results in 10 patients undergoing transseptal-crossed VE. These data highlight the fact that more complex reconstruction is associated with lower success rates, and these issues should be discussed with any patient with a history of prior inguinal surgery.[37]

Prior Vasectomy Reversal

Repeat vasectomy reversal is a valid option after failed initial reversal.[38] Hernandez and Sabanegh[39] performed a retrospective review of 41 men (38 had one previous reversal and 3 had multiple previous reversals) who underwent repeat vasectomy reversal. This group overall had a patency rate of 79% and a pregnancy rate of 31%. The only statistically significant predictor for successful pregnancy was a history of conception with the current partner. Pasquallotto and colleagues[40] reviewed 18 patients who underwent repeat VE. The overall patency rate was 66.7%. Patency rates varied according to the level of anastomosis: 66.7% in the caput, 62.5% in the corpus, and 100% in the cauda. Each of these studies indicates that failure of prior reconstruction is not a contraindication to reconstructive procedures. However, the lower pregnancy rates after VE should be discussed with the patient.

Same Partner

Outcomes of vasectomy reversal in men with the same female partners are better than those for men with new partners. The Vasovasostomy Study Group[1] first described this relationship (Table 1). Chan and Goldstein[6] confirmed this higher success rate in a subgroup of 27 men undergoing vasectomy reversal who had the same partner as before their vasectomy. They achieved a patency rate of 100% and a pregnancy rate of 86%. Interestingly, the live-birth rate in couples with the death of a child was 100%. Chan and Goldstein proposed previous proven fecundity as a couple, shorter obstructive interval, and stronger emotional dedication to having a child as possible reasons for higher success rates in men with same female partners.

Partner Age

As with any infertility intervention, the age of the female partner is an important factor in assessing the appropriateness of the intervention. Hinz and colleagues,[41] in a retrospective analysis of 212 patients undergoing vasectomy reversal, identified

Table 1
Same female partner is associated with higher pregnancy rates

Effect of Indication on Fertility After Vasovasostomy	
Indication	No. Pregnant/Total in Group (%)
Divorce	303/612 (50)
Death of child/same partner	16/21 (76)
Other	87/154 (57)

Modified from Belker AM, Thomas AJ, Fuchs EF, et al. Results of 1,469 microsurgical vasectomy reversals by the Vasovasostomy Group. J Urol 1991;145:507; with permission.

age of female partner greater than 40 years as a predictor for lower pregnancy rates compared to those 30 to 39 years or less than 30 years ($P = 0.014$ univariate and $P = 0.010$ multivariate). Gerrard and colleagues[42] described patency/pregnancy rates for patients with female partners aged 20 to 24, 25 to 29, 30 to 34, 35 to 39, and greater than 40 as 90%/67%, 89%/52%, 90%/57%, 86%/54%, and 83%/14%, respectively. The pregnancy rate for patients with female partners aged greater than 40 years was 14%, compared to 56% for those with female partners aged less than 40 years. These two studies indicate a precipitous drop in pregnancy rates when the female partner is greater than 40 years old.

IVF-ICSI is also greatly influenced by the age of the female partner. Reported overall pregnancy rates for IVF-ICSI is 36.9% in women less than 35 years old, compared to 10.7% in women greater than 40 years old.[24] IVF pregnancy rates in couples with only male-factor infertility are 44.7% in women less than 35 years old and 20.2% in women greater than 40 years old, indicating a detrimental effect of advanced partner age.[24] Fuchs and Burt[28] found a similar decline in pregnancy rates with advanced partner age that was seen in Gerrard and colleagues's study. They found pregnancy rates of 64% for those with female partners aged less than 30 years of age and pregnancy rates of 28% for those with female partners greater than 40 years of age. Their data suggest slightly better pregnancy rates with vasectomy reversal (28%) when compared to IVF-ICSI for only male-factor inferility (20.2%) in this subgroup of couples with females aged greater than 40 years.

Antisperm Antibodies

Although discussed as a factor that may affect successful outcome, assessment of antisperm antibodies (ASA) is not generally performed prior to proceeding with a vasectomy reversal.[43]

Meinertz and colleagues,[44] in an effort to suggest the importance of ASA testing before

vasectomy reversal, reported on 216 men who underwent VV and were subsequently tested with the mixed antiglobulin reaction for IgA and IgG specific to ASA bound to the sperm membrane. Free ASA in serum and seminal plasma were analyzed with the gelatin agglutination test and the tray agglutination test. In a subgroup with a pure IgG response, the rate of conception was 85.7%. In this group, only 42.9% of men who also had IgA on the sperm achieved pregnancy. When 100% of the sperm were covered with IgA, the pregnancy rate decreased to 21.7%. The combination of IgA on all sperm and a serum titer of greater than 255 was associated with a pregnancy rate of 0.

Carbone and colleagues[45] published a study of 14 patients with partial obstruction (epididymal fullness) and ASA who had previously undergone vasectomy reversal. All patients had positive ASA status as defined as greater than 20% binding on indirect immunobead assay testing. After repeat vasectomy reversal without treatment of the ASA, the pregnancy rate was 50%. Sperm motility increased from 4.4% to 52.3%, and sperm concentration doubled. This suggests the reason for failure of the first vasectomy reversal was technical and not from ASA. The investigators concluded that ASA status is not a significant factor in failed VVs.

ASA form in the vast majority of individuals subjected to vasectomy.[46] This fact, in conjunction with the fact that the majority of men will conceive after a technically successful vasectomy reversal, indicates the inability of ASA testing to predict successful vasectomy reversal. Therefore, determination of ASA status before attempted reversal is, in general, not recommended, as it will not affect the management of the individual patient.

INTRAOPERATIVE FACTORS
Surgeon Skill

Microsurgical reconstruction emphasizes technical skill and expertise. Outcomes improve with experience and refinement of technique. This was demonstrated in the fourfold greater success of VVs performed between 1994 and 1999, compared to those performed between 1980 and 1984, in a series from Holman and colleagues.[47]

VEs are technically more demanding, and some urologists offer only VV for vasectomy reversal. Chawla and colleagues[48] examined 22 cases of repeat vasectomy reversal after failed VV. Upon exploration, they found that 48% of the men had epididymal obstruction as the etiology for their initial failure. All surgeons offering vasectomy reversals should be able to offer VE if required, based on intraoperative findings.

There have been many attempts to train surgeons in new techniques using formal laboratory experiences. The authors performed a survey to assess the success of a group of urologists who had participated in a microsurgery course compared to those who had not (Nagler HM, Belker AM, unpublished data, 1997). Those surgeons who performed microsurgical VV without practice had a 53% patency rate, compared with an 89% patency rate for those surgeons who practiced their microsurgical skills in a laboratory before employing them clinically. This survey demonstrated the need to practice microsurgery in the laboratory before conducting it in a clinical setting.

Intravasal Fluid

The characteristics of the intravasal fluid and the presence of sperm in the fluid from the testicular vas deferens affect the likelihood of successful vasectomy reversal. Of patients with copious, clear fluid and motile intravasal sperm, 94% had a return of sperm to the ejaculate, compared with 60% of those with no sperm in the vasal fluid. The pregnancy rates for these two groups were 63% and 31%, respectively.[1]

The decision to proceed with VV or to convert to VE is based on intraoperative inspection of the intravasal fluid, epididymal findings, the patient's desires based on preoperative consultation, history of prior attempted VV, and the urologist's skills. Despite the widely held dogma based upon prior reports, Sharlip[49] reported a patency rate of 80% for patients without intravasal fluid at the time of VV. Nevertheless, most urologists believe that VV should be performed only if fluid containing whole sperm or sperm parts is encountered. Sigman[50] reported excellent patency rates of 95%, 100%, and 100% for patients with sperm heads, sperm with short tails, and whole sperm, respectively. This study answered an often debated issue and now enables the urologist to

perform the technically more successful procedure with the confidence that the results will be comparable for each of these observed findings. However, Kolettis and colleagues[51] demonstrated a patency/pregnancy rate of 76%/35% when only sperm parts were encountered. The patency rate improved to 84% if cases with an occasional sperm head were excluded. This success rate is not as good as when complete sperm are encountered, but it is at least as good as most urologists' experience with VE. VV is indicated when only sperm parts are encountered, but the urologist should consider VE if only an occasional sperm head is encountered.

If clear or copious fluid is encountered without sperm in the first-time reversal patient with an obstructive interval less than 11 years, VV may also be performed. Kolettis and colleagues[52] reported a patency/pregnancy rate of 80%/38% in this subgroup. However, after the obstructive interval exceeds 11 years, VE is recommended.

VE is indicated if intravasal fluid is absent or if it is a thick, inspissated, toothpaste-like fluid. The epididymis should be examined (not explored) when there is thick fluid without sperm or when no fluid is observed. If a clear epididymal obstruction is encountered, VE is generally indicated.

Testicular Remnant Length

Witt and colleagues[53] reported a correlation between the length of the postvasectomy testicular vasal remnant and the intravasal fluid characteristics: the longer the segment, the better the intravasal fluid. They showed that 94% of patients with a testicular remnant greater than 2.7 cm had whole sperm in the intravasal fluid. This observation has not been confirmed by other investigators, presumably because of the subjective nature of the measurement relative to the convoluted portion of the vas and that the length only predicted the intraoperative vasal findings. Preoperatively, one is unable to accurately assess the vasal remnant.

Sperm Granulomas

Sperm granulomas are discovered microscopically between 10% and 30% of the time in men undergoing vasectomy reversal. It is probable that, given sufficient time, all men will develop sperm granulomas at the vasectomy site, the epididymis, or the rete testis. Although sperm granulomas presumably allow the efferent ductules to vent into surrounding tissues, thus allowing the release of pressure that may protect the epididymis from tubule rupture or dysfunction, there was no difference in the technical or functional results achieved in patients with or without the presence of sperm granulomas. Sperm granulomas have been associated with better grades of sperm quality in the intraoperative vas; however, the Vasovasostomy Study Group found that a sperm granuloma at the site was not associated with successful repair. Patency/pregnancy rates were 96%/63% when a sperm granuloma was present bilaterally, and they were 85%/51% when it was absent bilaterally. These differences were not statistically significant.[1] Boorjian and colleagues[5] also could not demonstrate a statistically significant difference. However, Bolduc and colleagues[54] found an odds ratio (95% confidence interval) of 2.4 (1.3–4.4) and statistical significance (0.004) in favor of patients with sperm granulomas. More studies are required to evaluate the relationship between the presence of sperm granulomas and the rates of success.

Vasectomy Site and Length

The site of vasectomy may result in a greater technical challenge for repair if it is in the convoluted portion, as opposed to the straight portion, of the vas deferens. In their single surgeon series, Patel and Sigman[55] found patency rates of 98.1% and 97.3% for convoluted VV and straight VV, respectively, and this difference was not statistically significant. They conclude that although convoluted VV is considered technically more challenging, technical success is comparable with straight VV. However, this finding reflects only that single urologist's skill level and not that of all urologists performing microsurgical reconstruction.

Although not studied, when there is a long segment of vas absent from an "aggressive" vasectomy, reversal is technically more demanding and may result in tension on the anastomosis. A longer absent segment may also necessitate more vigorous mobilization of the vas with greater potential for devascularization and subsequent fibrosis.

POSTOPERATIVE MANAGEMENT

There is no uniform approach to the management of patients after vasectomy reversal. Issues that may have an impact on the ultimate results include a period of abstinence, avoidance of activity, and use of anti-inflammatory agents.

An informal survey of 12 microsurgeons was performed to determine the recommendations of these specialists.[56] The period of abstinence recommended by these experts varied from 2 to 4 weeks. Patients were instructed to avoid strenuous activity from 2 to 6 weeks. Only a few of those surveyed routinely used anti-inflammatory agents.

The impact of postoperative management on success has not been systematically studied.

ENSURING SUCCESS

Successful microsurgical vasectomy reversal may be attained by: (1) eliciting the relevant history, (2) the performance of the appropriate physical examination, (3) careful analysis of the intraoperative findings, and (4) appropriate postoperative management. Success rates can be maximized with appropriate training, practice, and experience. The patient and his partner should be appropriately apprised and have realistic expectations.

REFERENCES

1. Belker AM, Thomas AJ, Fuchs EF, et al. Results of 1,469 microsurgical vasectomy reversals by the Vasovasostomy Group. J Urol 1991;145:505–11.
2. Owen E, Kapila H. Vasectomy reversal. Review of 475 microsurgical vasovasostomies. Med J Aust 1984;140:398–400.
3. Silber SJ. Pregnancy after vasovasostomy for vasectomy reversal. A study of factors affecting long-term return of fertility in 282 patients followed for 10 years. Hum Reprod 1989;4:318–22.
4. Fox M. Vasectomy reversal—microsurgery for best results. Br J Urol 1994;73:449–53.
5. Boorjian S, Lipkin M, Goldstein M. The impact of obstructive interval and sperm granuloma on outcome of vasectomy reversal. J Urol 2004;171: 304–6.
6. Chan PT, Goldstein M. Superior outcomes of microsurgical vasectomy reversal in men with the same female partners. Fertil Steril 2004;81:1371–4.
7. McLoughlin MG. Vasoepididymostomy: the role of the microscope. Can J Surg 1982;25:41–3.
8. Dubin L, Amelar RD. Magnified surgery for epididymovasostomy. Urology 1984;23:525–8.
9. Fogdestam I, Fall M, Nilsson S. Microsurgical epididymovasostomy in the treatment of occlusive azoospermia. Fertil Steril 1986;46:925–9.
10. Lee HY. A 20-year experience with epididymovasostomy for pathologic epididymal obstruction. Fertil Steril 1987;47:487–91.
11. Fuchs EF. Restoring fertility through epididymovasostomy. Contemp Urol 1991;3:27–31.
12. Schlegel PN, Goldstein M. Microsurgical vasoepididymostomy: refinements and results. J Urol 1993; 150:1165–8.
13. Matsuda T, Horii Y, Muguruma K, et al. Microsurgical epididymovasostomy for obstructive azoospermia: factors affecting postoperative fertility. Eur Urol 1994;26:322–6.
14. Matthews GJ, Schlegel PN, Goldstein M. Patency following microsurgical vasoepididymostomy and

vasovasostomy: temporal considerations. J Urol 1995;154:2070–3.

15. Jarow JP, Sigman M, Buch JP, et al. Delayed appearance of sperm after end-to-side vasoepididymostomy. J Urol 1995;153:1156–8.

16. Boeckx W, Van Helden S. Microsurgical vasoepididymostomy in the treatment of occlusive azoospermia. Br J Urol 1996;77:577–9.

17. Kolettis PN, Thomas AJ Jr. Vasoepididymostomy for vasectomy reversal: a critical assessment in the era of intracytoplasmic sperm injection. J Urol 1997;158: 467–70.

18. Berardinucci D, Zini A, Jarvi K. Outcome of microsurgical reconstruction in men with suspected epididymal obstruction. J Urol 1998;159:831–4.

19. Berger RE. Triangulation end-to-side vasoepididymostomy. J Urol 1998;159:1951–3.

20. Hibi H, Yamada Y, Honda N, et al. Microsurgical vasoepididymostomy with sperm cryopreservation for future assisted reproduction. Int J Urol 2000;7: 435–9.

21. Marmar JL. Modified vasoepididymostomy with simultaneous double needle placement, tubulotomy and tubular invagination. J Urol 2000;163:483–6.

22. Schrepferman CG, Carson MR, Sparks AE, et al. Need for sperm retrieval and cryopreservation at vasectomy reversal. J Urol 2001;166:1787–9.

23. Schoor RA, Elhanbly SM, Ross LS, et al. The influence of obstructive interval on patency rates following microsurgical epididymovasostomy. World J Urol 2002;19:453–6.

24. Centers for Disease Control and Prevention. Assisted reproductive technology success rates: National Summary and Fertility Clinic Reports. Available at: http://www.cdc.gov/ART; 2005. Accessed January 25, 2009.

25. Kolettis PN, Sabanegh ES, D'amico AM, et al. Outcomes for vasectomy reversal performed after obstructive intervals of at least 10 years. Urology 2002;60:885–8.

26. Centers for Disease Control and Prevention. Assisted reproductive technology success rates: National Summary and Fertility Clinic Reports. Available at: http://www.cdc.gov/ART; 2002. Accessed January 25, 2009.

27. Malizia BA, Hacker MR, Penzias AS. Cumulative live-birth rates after in vitro fertilization. N Engl J Med 2009;360:236–43.

28. Fuchs EF, Burt RA. Vasectomy reversal performed 15 years or more after vasectomy: correlation of pregnancy outcome with partner age and with pregnancy results of in vitro fertilization with intracytoplasmic sperm injection. Fertil Steril 2002;77: 516–9.

29. Parekattil SJ, Kuang W, Agarwal A, et al. Model to predict if a vasoepididymostomy will be required for vasectomy reversal. J Urol 2005;173:1681–4.

30. Parekattil SK, Kuang W, Kolettis PN, et al. Multi-institutional validation of vasectomy reversal predictor. J Urol 2006;175:247–9.

31. Potts JM, Pasqualotto FF, Nelson D, et al. Patient characteristics associated with vasectomy reversal. J Urol 1999;161:1835–9.

32. Sigman M, Jarow JP. Endocrine evaluation of infertile men. Urology 1997;50:659–62.

33. Shin D, Lipshultz LI, Goldstein M, et al. Herniorrhaphy with polypropylene mesh causing inguinal vasal obstruction: a preventable cause of obstructive azoospermia. Ann Surg 2005;241:553–8.

34. Nagler HM, Belletete BA, Gerber E, et al. Laparoscopic retrieval of retroperitoneal vas deferens in vasovasostomy for postinguinal herniorrhaphy obstructive azoospermia. Fertil Steril 2005;83(6): 1842.

35. Lizza EF, Marmar JL, Schmidt SS, et al. Trans-septal crossed vasovasostomy. J Urol 1985;134:1131–2.

36. Sabanegh E Jr, Thomas AJ Jr. Effectiveness of crossover transseptal vasoepididymostomy in treating complex obstructive azoospermia. Fertil Steril 1995;63:392–5.

37. Thomas AJ, Sabenegh ES, Nagler HM. Complex reconstruction for obstruction of the vas deferens and epididymis. Atlas of surgical management of male infertility. Tokyo: Igaku-Shoin Medical Publishers Inc; 1995. p. 71.

38. Hollingsworth MR, Sandlow JI, Schrepferman CG, et al. Repeat vasectomy reversal yields high success rates. Fertil Steril 2007;88:217–9.

39. Hernandez J, Sabanegh ES. Repeat vasectomy reversal after initial failure. J Urol 1999;161:1153–6.

40. Pasqualotto FF, Agarwal A, Srivastava M, et al. Fertility outcome after repeat vasoepididymostomy. J Urol 1999;162:1626–8.

41. Hinz S, Rais-Bahrami S, Kempkensteffen C, et al. Fertility rates following vasectomy reversal: importance of age of the female partner. Urol Int 2008; 81:416–20.

42. Gerrard ER Jr, Sandlow JI, Oster RA, et al. Effect of female partner age on pregnancy rates after vasectomy reversal. Fertil Steril 2007;87:1340–4.

43. Linnet L, Hjort T, Fogh-Andersen P. Association between failure to impregnate after vasovasostomy and sperm agglutinins in semen. Lancet 1981;1: 117–9.

44. Meinertz H, Linnet L, Fogh-Andersen P, et al. Antisperm antibodies and fertility after vasovasostomy: a follow-up study of 216 men. Fertil Steril 1990;64:315–8.

45. Carbone DJ, Shah A, Thomas AJ Jr, et al. Partial obstruction, not antisperm antibodies, causing infertility after vasovasostomy. J Urol 1998;159:827–30.

46. Haas GG Jr. Antibody mediated causes of male infertility. Urol Clin North Am 1987;14:539–50.

47. Holman CDJ, Wisniewski ZS, Semmens JB, et al. Population-based outcomes after 28,246 in-hospital

vasectomies and 1902 vasovasostomies in Western Australia. Br J Urol 2000;86:1043–9.

48. Chawla A, O'Brien J, Lisi M, et al. Should all urologists performing vasectomy reversal be able to perform vasoepididymostomies if required? J Urol 2004;172:829–30.

49. Sharlip I. Absence of fluid during vasectomy reversal has no prognostic significance. J Urol 1996;155: 365–9.

50. Sigman M. The relationship between intravasal sperm quality and patency rates after vasovasostomy. J Urol 2004;171:307–9.

51. Kolettis PN, Burns JR, Nangia AK, et al. Outcomes for vasovasostomy performed when only sperm parts are present in the vasal fluid. J Androl 2006; 27:565–7.

52. Kolettis PN, D'Amico AM, Box L, et al. Outcomes for vasovaostomy with bilateral intravasal azoospermia. J Androl 2003;24:22–4.

53. Witt MA, Heron S, Lipshultz LI. The postvasectomy length of testicular remnant: a predictor of surgical outcome in microscopic vasectomy reversal. J Urol 1994;151:892–4.

54. Bolduc S, Fischer MA, Deceunick G, et al. Factors predicting overall success: a review of 74 microsurgical vasovasostomies. Can Urol Assoc J 2007;1:388–91.

55. Patel SR, Sigman R. Comparison of outcomes of vasovasostomy performed in the convoluted and straight vas deferens. J Urol 2008;179:256.

56. Nagler HM, Rotman M. Predictive parameters for microsurgical reconstruction. Urol Clin North Am 2002;29:913–9.

Cost-Effectiveness of Vasectomy Reversal

Paul Robb, MD[a], Jay I. Sandlow, MD[a,b],*

KEYWORDS
- Vasectomy reversal • Obstructive azoospermia
- Sperm retrieval • IVF • Infertility

In the modern era of in vitro fertilization (IVF), the options for couples who have obstructive azoospermia (OA) have improved tremendously. With the advent and improvement of intracytoplasmic sperm injection (ICSI), couples who previously had limited choices for conceiving after a vasectomy (eg, vasectomy reversal [VR] or donor sperm) now may have a simple sperm retrieval (SR) in conjunction with IVF in order to achieve a biologic pregnancy. With these techniques many centers are reporting success rates of more than 50% per cycle and, although the cost of treatment tends to be higher than with surgical reconstruction, IVF provides a realistic alterative. In this era of cost-consciousness and containment, however, and limited health care resources for much of the population, it is important to examine all the factors and consequences that are involved with both surgical reconstruction as well as SR/IVF/ICSI. Many factors need to be considered when making a decision and there are no randomized controlled studies to use for guidance. Factors to consider include risks for procedures, cost-effectiveness, number of children desired, female fertility issues (including taking into account the time to conceive after VR), and future contraception needs.

This article examines these factors, presents the advantages and disadvantages of each approach, and suggests situations where one modality may be superior to another.

SURGICAL RECONSTRUCTION FOR OBSTRUCTIVE AZOOSPERMIA

The most common cause of OA is vasectomy, although there are infectious, congenital, traumatic, and idiopathic causes. The two types of repair, vasovasostomy (VV) and vasoepididymostomy (EV), are described in detail elsewhere.[1] Typically, patency and pregnancy rates are higher for VV than EV, and these rates are surgeon specific. Most series report patency rates of greater than 85% for VV and approximately 60% to 70% for EV, with variable pregnancy outcomes.[2,3] The cost for VR varies based on surgeons' fees, operative costs, and anesthesia fees. It is important for patients and providers to compare real costs and success rates specific to their situations rather than generalized costs that may not reflect the local marketplace. This is true for surgical reconstruction and IVF.

SPERM RETRIEVAL WITH IN VITRO FERTILIZATION/INTRACYTOPLASMIC SPERM INJECTION

As success rates for IVF have improved, the use of this technique has increased. As more programs are becoming adept at working with testicular and epididymal sperm, the success rates for SR/IVF/ICSI have improved dramatically without a significant rise in costs. This has led to improved cost-effectiveness for this procedure. Furthermore, as pregnancy rates have risen, the number of embryos transferred has declined, leading to a smaller number of multiple gestation pregnancies.[4] As several investigators have reported, however, the success rate of SR/IVF/ICSI must approach unrealistically high percentages in order to counteract the significant difference in cost as compared to VR.[5]

a Department of Obstetrics and Gynecology, Medical College of Wisconsin, 9200 West Wisconsin Avenue, Milwaukee, WI 53226, USA
b Department of Urology, Medical College of Wisconsin, 9200 West Wisconsin Avenue, Milwaukee, WI 53226, USA
* Corresponding author.
E-mail address: jsandlow@mcw.edu (J.I. Sandlow).

Urol Clin N Am 36 (2009) 391–396
doi:10.1016/j.ucl.2009.05.003

In order to fully understand the factors related to success, one must be somewhat familiar with the IVF procedure. IVF involves the use of exogenous gonadotropins to bring about multifollicular growth. After monitoring the growth and maturation of the follicles, the oocytes are retrieved though an ultrasound-guided transvaginal percutaneous puncture and aspiration of the follicles. In the case of obstructive azoospermia, the retrieved sperm are used for ICSI to fertilize the eggs. The resultant embryos, typically on day 3 or 5 after oocyte retrieval, then are transferred into the woman's uterus. The number of embryos placed in the uterus varies with different institutions and usually takes into account the female partner's age and the embryo quality along with success or failure from any previous cycles. Fortunately, pregnancy with ICSI has been shown to be possible with spermatozoa from almost any source, including testis, epididymis, vas deferens, and the ejaculate, so that the success of assisted reproductive technology (ART) essentially relates mainly to female factors (female infertility issues, age, and oocyte quality and quantity). The single greatest prognostic factor for IVF success is the age of the female partner. With the increasing success of the IVF procedure, there has been an emphasis of late on considering single embryo transfers as a means of avoiding the complications and costs of multiple pregnancies. As a result of lower per-cycle pregnancy rates with single versus multiple embryo transfers and because most of the cost of ART is not covered by insurance, this push has not translated into routine practice. Risks for the IVF process that need to be considered include the risk for multiples and their complications,[6] injuries as a result of stimulation or oocyte retrieval,[7] ovarian hyperstimulation syndrome,[8] and the slight elevation in congenital anomalies.[9]

FEMALE FACTORS

Several studies have examined female partner age as a predictor of VR success. Gerrard and colleagues[10] examined success rates of VRs in 294 patients and pregnancy rates for various female partner ages. They found pregnancy rates above 50% in the age categories below age 40 but only 14% in those couples in which the female partner was over age 40. They concluded that couples in which the female partner is over age 40 should have careful preoperative counseling about their chance for pregnancy, whether or not they choose VR or IVF. Silber and Grotjan[11] summarized their data on 1735 patients who could be contacted out of a total of 4010 patients who underwent VR and found that the one factor that

had the most significant impact on pregnancy rate was the age of the female partner. They reported pregnancy rates of over 90% when the female partner was under age 30 but less than 55% when the female partner was over age 40. Another finding to consider from this study was that 23% of the pregnancies did not occur until more than 2 years after VR. These 2 years may be enough to cause a significant diminution in female partner reproductive potential, commonly referred to as ovarian reserve (discussed later).

The Society for Assisted Reproductive Technology's (SART) data highlight the importance of female partner age when considering ART. When examining the literature, however, it is important to realize that in all age groups, ART success has been improving steadily since its inception. Due to this improvement over time, it is imperative that one consider the year in which a study reports the ART success it is using to compare with VR, if one is to make a meaningful comparison. A study by Deck and colleagues[12] used a result of 8% for the live birth rate in women over age 36, based on the results of a 1997 study group, to conclude that vasectomy was still cost effective in couples with an older female partner. Physicians must consider not only the rates for ART success quoted in any given study and the year it was written but also the rates in their own center or the center to which they refer patients to decide if the results for a study population can be extrapolated to their patient population. An examination of the SART national numbers for the year 2006, for cycles that include only male factor, shows that pregnancy rates range from a high of 49% (women aged <35), to 41% (ages 35–37), to 30% (ages 38–40), to 19% (ages 41–42), and to 13% (ages 43–44). These numbers are not exclusive to VR but include all male factors. It is presumed that the majority of patients undergoing a vasectomy have previously proved male fertility potential, so these data may underestimate the success of ART in this subset of male infertility. Hsieh[13] used Markov modeling, a form of decision analysis in which a hypothetical patient proceeds through health states over time based on predefined probabilities and costs. When considering cost, physicians need to consider both partners when comparing VR with SR/IVF. The authors concluded that ART yields a higher pregnancy rate but does so at a higher cost than does VR. When the authors performed a sensitivity analysis to determine which variables had an impact on the Markov model, they found that female partner age had a greater effect on cost-effectiveness than did the obstructive interval. Many cost analysis studies suggest that, particularly in couples with a younger female partner who have no other fertility issues, VR is more cost effective (**Table 1**). However, due to the excellent ART success rates in this population, couples who desire only one child might prefer ART over VR. If the couple does opt for ART in this situation, then a single embryo transfer should also be strongly considered. The 2006 SART data also showed a 32% twin and 2% triplet or higher order

Table 1
Comparison of cost-effectiveness studies for vasectomy reversal versus sperm retrieval/in vitro fertilization

Author (Year)	Study Design	More Cost-Effective VR Versus SR/IVF	Comments
Pavlovich (1997)[14]	Model	VR	VR pregnancy rates based on six fellowship-trained urologists; IVF pregnancy rates based on average of four different IVF centers.
Kolettis (1997)[15]	Retrospective case review	VR	All VR were EV. Conclusions based on IVF pregnancy rate of only 29%.
Donovan et al (1998)[5]	Retrospective case review	VR	All VR were redo procedures; IVF pregnancy rate high, but SR costs were same as VR costs.
Deck & Berger (2000)[12]	Retrospective case review	VR	IVF pregnancy rates extremely low (8%) for women >36 y of age.
Heidenreich et al (2000)[16]	Retrospective case review	VR	Based on IVF pregnancy rates from 1998.
Garceau et al (2002)[17]	Review	VR	Based on four studies, all retrospective.
Pasqualotto (2004)[18]	Review	VR if <15 y SR/IVF if >15 y or female factor	—
Meng et al (2005)[19]	Decision modeling	VR if patency >80%; SR/IVF if patency <80%	Used computer-generated model and algorithm.
Hsieh et al (2007)[13]	Markov modeling	VR if WTP <$65K; SR/IVF if WTP >$65K	Based on WTP. At higher rates of WTP, female age has less impact, favors IVF.
Lee et al (2008)[20]	Decision analysis model	VR	VR success rates based on six high-volume centers; IVF success rates based on five high volume centers; indirect costs also factored into analysis.

Abbreviations: EV, vasoepididymostomy; SR/IVF, sperm retrieval/in vitro fertilization; VR, vasectomy reversal; WTP, willingness to pay.

multiple rate with ART in the under age 35 group with an average of 2.3 embryos transferred. In the over age 38 group, Hsieh's Markov modeling suggests that ART may be more cost effective than VR, although some of this also is dependent on the time from vasectomy. What about those in the group that is over age 42? With either treatment they are going to have a low likelihood of success. Would this group be better off with the low probability but also lower cost option of VR to have at least some chance to conceive? There are no trials to guide the decision process. In this case, it is important to counsel such couples on the better pregnancy success option of using donor eggs and the high rate of aneuploidy in any conceptions using the female partner's own eggs.[21] As in the Silber study, it is usual to present VR pregnancy rates as cumulative rates over time and not per month whereas IVF success usually is reported as per month as represented per cycle. This is in part because of the one-time cost of the VR whereas IVF treatment incurs costs with each cycle. This does not make for an entirely fair comparison, however. Malizia and colleagues[22] retrospectively studied 6164 patients undergoing 14,248 cycles and analyzed cumulative success rates with IVF. These patients went through up to 6 cycles with a mean of 2.3 cycles. Success again varied with female partner age. Among patients who were younger than 35 years of age, the live birth rates (not just pregnancy) after six cycles were 86% (optimistic calculation) and 65% (conservative calculation). Among patients who were 40 years of age or older, the corresponding rates were 42% (optimistic) and 23% (conservative). The differences between the optimistic and conservative calculations relates to how dropouts were handled. These numbers are in the same range as Silber's, which allowed for a much longer follow-up time period. The Malizia study was done in a state that has mandated IVF coverage and for most patients, in nonmandated states, the cost of 6 cycles would be prohibitive. The mean number of cycles, however, was less than 2.5. They also noted that their pregnancy and live birth rates were lower than the national average for 2005 (date for completion of the study). For women under age 35, they reported a first-cycle live birth rate of 33%, which is slightly lower than the live birth rate per cycle start (all starts, not only first starts) of 37% reported by SART for women under age 35 for 2005. They may, therefore, underestimate the cumulative pregnancy rates expected with ART. The Markov modeling by Hseih (discussed previously) also showed that with increasing willingness to pay (WTP), ART was more cost effective over a wider range of female partner age. It must, therefore, be factored in how much a couple can pay and how long, for both medical and social reasons, can they wait.

OVARIAN RESERVE TESTING

Related to age is the concept of ovarian reserve, which can be viewed as an imprecise measure of a woman's reproductive potential. There are many tests for this that have been proposed, including a day 3 follicle-stimulating hormone (FSH) level, a clomiphene citrate challenge test (CCCT), inhibin levels, antimüllerian hormone levels, and antral follicle counts. All show less than 100% sensitivity or specificity[23] but are used as guides for success with ART. Scott and colleagues[24] used life table analysis to follow 589 couples for 45 months to study pregnancy rates over different age categories in those who had normal and abnormal CCCT results undergoing a variety of fertility treatment options. Although pregnancies did occur in those who had an abnormal CCCT, they occurred at a much lower rate and this effect was exacerbated in older patients. It would seem prudent to use some established measure of ovarian reserve, such as a CCCT, on the female partner prior to proceeding with a VR or IVF to help guide the counseling of patients. This may be even more important in female patients over age 35 to take advantage of the shortened time to pregnancy with ART, as ovarian reserve only worsens with time, and this is especially salient if there are already signs of diminished ovarian reserve.

STUDIES COMPARING COST-EFFECTIVENESS

Various studies have examined cost in decision analysis modeling.[17] Lee and colleagues,[20] factoring in the costs of procedures, indirect costs of complications, lost productivity, and multiple gestations, found that VR seemed more cost effective than SR/IVF/ISCI. They calculated a cost per pregnancy in 2005 for a VR at $20,903 compared with a cost of $54,797 for testicular sperm extraction (TESE) and $56,861 for microscopic epididymal sperm aspiration (MESA) when the latter two are combined with IVF. They concluded that VR was more cost effective than percutaneous TESE or MESA. They did not factor in, however, costs of future contraception in those who underwent a reversal of a highly effective contraceptive method nor did they consider the impact of female partner age. Hsieh's Markov modeling concluded that ART yields a higher pregnancy rate but does so at a higher cost than does

VR. Lee and colleagues[18] examined the cost-effectiveness of VR based on the type of procedure performed. They modeled costs per pregnancy based on patency rates of VR and various pregnancy rates for VR and IVF. The investigators demonstrated that if the expected patency rate was greater than 80%, VR was likely to be more cost effective than SR/IVF, regardless of the pregnancy rate. Conversely, if the expected patency rate was less than 80%, SR/IVF was more cost-effective, regardless of the pregnancy rate. These data help clinicians counsel couples based on the expected outcome of a VR. For example, in a patient who has an obstructive interval of greater than 15 years, the likelihood of the need for EV is high, thus lowering the expected patency rate.[25]

One of the main difficulties in comparing cost-effectiveness of VR and SR/IVF/ICSI is the lack of randomized or controlled trials. Most studies are biased from the outset and only examine couples who have chosen their route of treatment based on various factors. When examining the reported success rates in many of these studies, it becomes apparent that treatment often is directed towards the perceived "higher" success rate, thus skewing the data. For example, in a study that compared the effectiveness of VV versus SR/IVF/ICSI from Germany, the pregnancy rate for VV was 58% with an average obstructive interval of 7.8 years and a cost per live birth of 2793 €. This is in line with many reported studies of VV outcome. The pregnancy rate for the couples undergoing IVF is only 20%, however, which is significantly lower than the rates reported for many centers, resulting in a cost per live birth of 14,547 €.[16] Furthermore, the costs for SR vary greatly and may artificially inflate the total cost of IVF treatment. Several studies report SR costs that are more than the cost of a VR. Most of these studies are older and used MESA, a technique that requires an operating room, advanced equipment, and typically an anesthesiologist. Many centers have moved towards percutaneous sperm retrieval methods, such as testicular sperm aspiration (TESA), however, which is typically performed in an office under local anesthesia, greatly reducing costs. It is incumbent on patients and practitioners to take all these variables into consideration when making comparisons (see **Table 1**). Most of the older studies favor VR, whereas the more recent studies show situations in which SR/IVF may be more cost effective.

Many factors need to be considered when counseling couples in whom the male partner has had a vasectomy. Most importantly, the male must not be considered in isolation but fertility must be considered as the result of an interaction between both partners in the couple. Beyond the technical aspects of VR, the following should be addressed: the risks and costs of alternative procedures; any female partner fertility issues, including ovarian reserve and the likelihood that this will change over the expected time to conceive naturally after a VR; how many children the couple desire; and, finally, what will be the couple's future contraceptive wishes.

LIMITATIONS AND CONSIDERATIONS

- In situations where pregnancy rates are low, the less-expensive treatment may be superior due to low likelihood of success of either treatment (older woman, elevated FSH, and so forth).
- In cases where time to conception is important (women over age 35, diminished ovarian reserve, and so forth), IVF may represent a faster alternative. Because pregnancy rates are lower in this situation, however, VR allows for multiple attempts over time.
- Each institution has its own biases in terms of treatment preference, costs, outcomes, and so forth. These must be taken into consideration when making recommendations.
- Patient preference is an important factor. Despite the lower cost of VR, some couples do not want to deal with repeat sterilization after they are finished having children. Other couples do not want the potential burden of caring for twins. Finally, some couples view the ability to conceive naturally as a deciding factor. Each of these issues must be discussed with couples and contributes to making a final decision.

SUMMARY

In this era of cost-consciousness and containment, it is imperative to examine not only treatment outcomes but also the cost of these treatments. With improvements in IVF outcomes and the continued development of less-invasive sperm retrieval methods, physicians and couples must examine all options available to the couple who has had surgical sterilization. VR remains the gold standard of treatment for most of these couples; however, certain situations may be present (eg, significant female factor or social factors) in which SR/IVF may be a better option for these couples. It is a physician's responsibility to present all of the options, along with the pros and cons of each, including cost, in order to help arrive at an informed decision.

REFERENCES

1. Lipshultz LI, Thomas AJ,Jr., Khera M. Procedures to improve sperm delivery: vasectomy reversal and vasoepididymostomy. In: Editor Wein, A. Campbell's urology 9th (edition Volume 1, Chapter) Philadelphia, WB Saunders; 2007.

2. Belker AM, Thomas AJ, Fuchs EF, et al. Results of 1,469 microsurgical vasectomy reversals by the Vasovasostomy Study Group. J Urol 1991;145:505–11.

3. Schiff J, Chan P, Li P, et al. Outcome and late failures compared in 4 techniques of microsurgical vasoepididymostomy in 153 consecutive men. J Urol 2005; 174:651–5.

4. 2008 compendium of practice committee reports. Fertil Steril 2008;90:S163–4.

5. Donovan JF Jr, DiBaise M, Sparks AE, et al. Comparison of microscopic epididymal sperm aspiration and intracytoplasmic sperm injection/in-vitro fertilization with repeat microscopic reconstruction following vasectomy: is second attempt vas reversal worth the effort? Hum Reprod 1998;13:387–93.

6. Van Voorhis BJ. Outcomes from assisted reproductive technology. Obstet Gynecol. 2006;107(1):183–200.

7. Maxwell KN, Cholst IN, Rosenwaks Z. The incidence of both serious and minor complications in young women undergoing oocyte donation. Fertil Steril 2008;90:2165–71.

8. Aboulghar MA, Mansour RT. Ovarian hyperstimulation syndrome: classifications and critical analysis of preventive measures. Hum Reprod Update 2003;9:275–89.

9. Shiota K, Yamada S. Assisted reproductive technologies and birth defects in child born through the IVF process. Congenit Anom (Kyoto) 2005;45(2):39–43.

10. Gerrard ER Jr, Sandlow JI, Oster RA, et al. Effect of female partner age on pregnancy rates after vasectomy reversal. Fertil Steril 2007;87:1340–4.

11. Silber SJ, Grotjan HE. Microscopic vasectomy reversal 30 years later: a summary of 4010 cases by the same surgeon. J Androl 2004;25:845–59.

12. Deck AJ, Berger RE. Should vasectomy reversal be performed in men with older female partners? J Urol 2000;163(1):105–6.

13. Hsieh MH, Meng MV, Turek PJ. Markov modeling of vasectomy reversal and ART for infertility: how do obstructive interval and female partner age influence cost effectiveness? Fertil Steril 2007;88:840–6.

14. Pavlovich CP, Schlegel PN. Fertility options after vasectomy: a cost-effectiveness analysis. Fertil Steril 1997;67:133–41.

15. Kolettis PN, Thomas AJ Jr. Vasoepididymostomy for vasectomy reversal: a critical assessment in the era of intracytoplasmic sperm injection. J Urol 1997;158: 467–70.

16. Heidenreich A, Altmann P, Engelmann UH. Microsurgical vasovasostomy versus microsurgical epididymal sperm aspiration/testicular extraction of sperm combined with intracytoplasmic sperm injection. A cost-benefit analysis. Eur Urol 2000;37(5): 609–14.

17. Garceau L, Henderson J, Davis LJ, et al. Economic implications of assisted reproductive techniques: a systematic review. Hum Reprod 2002;17(12): 3090–109.

18. Pasqualotto FF, Lucon AM, Sobreiro BP, et al. The best infertility treatment for vasectomized men: assisted reproduction or vasectomy reversal? Rev Hosp Clin Fac Med Sao Paulo 2004;59:312–5.

19. Meng MV, Greene KL, Turek PJ. Surgery or assisted reproduction? A decision analysis of treatment costs in male infertility. J Urol 2005;174:1926–31.

20. Lee R, Li PS, Schlegel PN, et al. Reassessing reconstruction in the management of obstructive azoospermia: reconstruction or sperm acquisition? Urol Clin North Am 2008;35(2):289–301.

21. Tarlatzis BC, Zepiridis L. Perimenopausal conception. Ann N Y Acad Sci 2003;997:93–104.

22. Malizia BA, Hacker MR, Penzias AS. Cumulative live-birth rates after in vitro fertilization. N Engl J Med 2009;360:236–43.

23. Broekmans FJ, Kwee J, Hendriks DJ, et al. A systematic review of tests predicting ovarian reserve and IVF outcome. Hum Reprod Update 2006;12(6): 685–718.

24. Scott RT, Opsahl MS, Leonardi MR, et al. Life table analysis of pregnancy rates in a general infertility population relative to ovarian reserve and patient age. Hum Reprod 1995;10:1706–10.

25. Parekattil SJ, Kuang W, Agarwal A, et al. Model to predict if a vasoepidimostomy will be required for vasectomy reversal. J Urol 2005;173(5):1681–4.

Index

Note: Page numbers of article titles are in **boldface** type.

Urol Clin N Am 36 (2009) 397–401
doi:10.1016/S0094-0143(09)00062-7

Moving?

Make sure your subscription moves with you!

To notify us of your new address, find your **Clinics Account Number** (located on your mailing label above your name), and contact customer service at:

E-mail: elspcs@elsevier.com

800-654-2452 (subscribers in the U.S. & Canada)
314-453-7041 (subscribers outside of the U.S. & Canada)

Fax number: 314-523-5170

Elsevier Periodicals Customer Service
11830 Westline Industrial Drive
St. Louis, MO 63146

*To ensure uninterrupted delivery of your subscription, please notify us at least 4 weeks in advance of move.

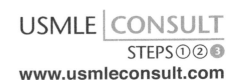

Printed and bound by CPI Group (UK) Ltd, Croydon, CR0 4YY

03/10/2024

01040344-0017